PREVENTION PLANNING IN MENTAL HEALTH

Sage Studies in Community Mental Health 9

SAGE STUDIES IN COMMUNITY MENTAL HEALTH

Series Editor
RICHARD H. PRICE
Community Psychology Program, University of Michigan

SAGE STUDIES IN COMMUNITY MENTAL HEALTH is a book series consisting of both single-authored and co-authored monographs and concisely edited collections of original articles which deal with issues and themes of current concern in the community mental health and related fields. Drawing from research in a variety of disciplines, the series seeks to link the work of the scholar and practitioner in this field, as well as advance the state of current knowledge in community mental health.

Volumes in this series:

Additional Volumes in Preparation

Prevention Planning in Mental Health

edited by

Jared
Hermalin

Jonathan A.
Morell

Volume 9, Sage Studies in Community Mental Health

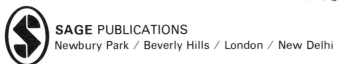

SAGE PUBLICATIONS
Newbury Park / Beverly Hills / London / New Delhi

For information address:

SAGE Publications, Inc.
2111 West Hillcrest Drive
Newbury Park, California 91320

SAGE Publications Inc.   SAGE Publications Ltd.
275 South Beverly Drive   28 Banner Street
Beverly Hills   London EC1Y 8QE
California 90212   England

SAGE PUBLICATIONS India Pvt. Ltd.
M-32 Market
Greater Kailash I
New Delhi 110 048 India

Printed in the United States of America

Library of Congress Cataloging-in-Publication Data

Main entry under title:

Prevention planning in mental health.

   (Sage studies in community mental health; v. 9)
   Includes bibliographical references.
   1. Mental health planning.   2. Mental illness—
Prevention.   3. Mental health planning—United States.
4. Preventive health services—United States—Planning.
I. Hermalin, Jared.   II. Morell, Jonathan A., 1946-
III. Series. [DNLM: 1. Mental Disorders—prevention &
control.   2. Mental Health Services—organization &
administration.   3. Preventive Health Services—
organization & administration.   W1 SA126M v.9 /
WM 30 P9435]
RA790.5.P68   1986   362.2   86-3874
ISBN 0-8039-2254-X

Contents

Series Editor's Preface

Interest in prevention has been expanding rapidly in recent years. In mental health, as in other fields, professionals are eager to identify viable prevention models and implement them in a wide range of community settings. Developing effective prevention programs is an important and exciting new challenge in the field of mental health. Furthermore, the field of prevention is now on the threshhold of moving from hopeful statements about the possibility of prevention in mental health to the less glamorous, but ultimately more important, task of generating sound evidence for the effectiveness of a wide range of different programs. This volume makes an important contribution to the move in that second critical stage in the development of preventive intervention in the field of mental health.

This volume is addressed to the planning of preventive programs. It begins by focusing on the conceptual and organizational activities that are critical to the sound implementation of effective prevention programs. In the opening chapter a general conceptual model for planning preventive programs describes the major functions of planning: need analysis, program justification, consensus building, and the development of information and evaluation systems. But there are unique opportunities and problems associated with planning prevention programs. The planning progress must take into account the fact that prevention programs are targeted to masses of individuals or populations, that timing is a critical factor in developing effective preventive interventions, requiring that we think in terms of extending time frames, and that mental health is not a neutral term, but one that is viewed differently by different constituencies of program recipients and sanctioners.

The editors have chosen their chapters well, addressing a wide range of arenas for prevention planning, sometimes focusing on vulnerable populations such as the aging, and in other cases focusing on settings including schools and the workplace. The chapters range from local to large-scale efforts at the federal level and also consider both formal organizational settings, such as the workplace, and less formal settings such as self-help groups. Each of these topical areas represents an important set of opportunities for the planning, development, and the implementation of prevention programs.

For the interested planner, the chapters in this volume have other desirable features. Each begins with a conceptual model in which the planning process is framed. At the same time, each chapter discusses numerous practical and concrete steps that are important to the successful implementation of any prevention program.

I am pleased to recommend this volume not only to mental health experts who are interested in the planning function but also to planners who are interested in mental health. It will be used by a wide range of professionals including nurses, social workers, psychologists, and sociologists. This book marks another step in transforming prevention efforts in mental health from a hope into a reality.

—*Richard H. Price*
University of Michigan

Chapter 1

PLANNING IN PREVENTION
Implications from a
General Model

JONATHAN A. MORELL

Each chapter in this book describes specific issues relevant to developing different types of prevention programs in mental health. As an introduction to those specifics, this chapter will address the interaction between generic aspects of planning and certain unique characteristics of prevention. This is an approach I have used successfully in analyzing the evaluation of prevention programs in mental health (Morell 1981). I am pleased to have this opportunity to extend my analysis to the more general activity of program planning.

Any planning process involves a set of discrete skills that must be applied whether one is working on prevention in mental health, a suspension bridge, or a research study. The case of prevention in mental health, however, has unique characteristics that make it difficult to apply those generic planning skills. The purpose of this chapter is to demonstrate that this is the case, and to sensitize readers to anticipate difficulties. I will present this case in three parts: (1) a discussion of the generic aspects of planning, (2) an explanation of the unique characteristics of prevention in mental health, and (3) a demonstration of the interaction between the general aspects of planning and the unique aspects of prevention.

THE NATURE OF PLANNING

Planners must, to some degree at least, exercise five sets of skills: need analysis, program justification, consensus building, program design, and information systems and evaluation.

Need Analysis

Need for a program is no guarantee of funding, nor may it even be the determining factor in a funding decision. Too many other factors intervene—value disagreements as to what constitutes need, differing views as to what needs are most important, institutional arrangements that are more conducive to some types of activities than others, and regulations governing the use of money for specific purposes. "Need" in some absolute sense may pale into insignificance in the face of these other factors. On the other hand, no program will ever begin unless a sympathetic party is convinced of the need for it. Nor can a program make it over the hurdles of funding and implementation without an ongoing ability to demonstrate need.

Need must be demonstrated on three levels. The first is in terms of the number of individuals who may receive a service. The second is the importance of the service to those who receive it. The third is the impact of the service on people and institutions involved with service recipients. As an example, consider the case of a health promotion program. There may be many people who can avoid health problems through such programs. The problems they avoid may be serious. Participation in the program may raise a company's productivity and decrease its health benefit costs. It is hard to imagine instituting a health promotion program unless a good case can be made for its need on each of these three levels.

Program Justification

Related to the assessment of need is the necessity of proposing a meaningful estimate of advantage. Although money is a favorite metric for such estimates, most people would agree that it is by no means the only metric. Cost effectiveness analysis, for instance, assumes the possibility of comparisons of output to effort without necessarily attaching a dollar value to the output. Values clarification efforts assume that one can determine what is important in personal or ethical terms. In this regard planners need two skills. The first is to ascertain what language of program justification will be salient to various groups. The second is to provide justification in the proper terms.

Consensus Building

Any new program faces the challenge of finding a way to fit into established organizational and cultural procedures. One aspect of the problem relates to agreement concerning what should be done to a specific population. Consider the development of a new vaccine for a previously unpreventable communicable disease. That development takes place against a social backdrop that includes

- general agreement that disease is not just an individual problem but, rather, a social problem because of its harmful effects when transmitted throughout the population;
- a set of professionals trained and willing to manufacture and administer the vaccine;
- a set of policymakers generally inclined to believe that vaccination is cost effective and free of significant health hazards;
- a population generally sympathetic to beliefs that biological scientists can develop and test effective drugs.

Contrast the vaccine case with an effort to institute social competency training in school systems or in children's psychological clinics.

- Is there agreement as to which professionals should provide the service?
- Will policymakers be inclined to accept the program?
- Is the general population likely to believe that such training is a good idea?

In all likelihood the answer to all of these questions will be "no." For all but the most traditional programs, planning must include a powerful effort to build a social and political consensus for the innovation. Absent such an agreement, few innovative programs will succeed.

Once a social consensus is built, one can go about the effort of getting money allocated. Two issues are important here. The first is the normal and ubiquitous competition for resources that is inevitable in any political endeavor. A second important issue may be the structure of funding mechanisms. In many cases the problem is not that money is unavailable, but rather that available money cannot be spent. Consider a health insurance policy that does not define certain mental health services as a reimbursable expense, or a nutrition program with an arguable definition of who needs supplemental assistance, or a medical services program that has no mandate to provide educational services. In all of these cases, building a consensus goes beyond getting people to agree that money should be spent. Rather, a consensus must also be built concerning legislation, regulation, and organizational structure.

In sum, those who wish to plan successfully must think in terms of building support in three realms: the general social context of the program, the legislative/regulatory/historical structure of services, and the availability of funds.

Program Design

How should a program be constructed? What services? What types of personnel? How many personnel? Where should the program be administered? How often? What mechanisms should be used to ensure a client base? What support services will be needed? A prerequisite to answering these questions is a well-articulated theory of program action—a theory that will help the planner specify who the program is most likely to help, the circumstances under which it can achieve its goals, and the extent of certainty that can be attached to achieving those goals.

Once this theory is specified it becomes possible to ascertain precisely how a program should be structured, what it should do, and how it should operate. Then one can address the more tangible challenges of planning—costing, allocation of non-monetary resources, and program management. *Costing* refers only to dollars—what money is needed, and how it should be spent? (There are also the additional problems related to constraints imposed by funding cycles and line item categories.) *Resource allocation* refers to coordinating all of the program elements that do not exist as dollars in an account. Volunteer time, contributed space in a building, donated advertising, free access to a computer system, and the like. All of these have a dollar value, but they cannot be exchanged one for the other. It may also be more difficult to use nonmonetary resources strictly according to one's own timetable. Thus in the planning process one must consider both the amount of resources available and the interrelationships that may exist among noninterchangeable resources.

Regarding *program management,* whether or not planners are themselves managers, they must consider issues related to management. Planners set goals, structure budgets, determine service locations, and engage in a host of other activities that set the basic constraints and options of all program personnel. Thus in the planning stage it is critical to conceptualize how a program will actually run, and to structure that program in a way that will promote successful management. Consider the all too common situation where a program's planners have set unrealistically high goals for the outcomes of the program. This situation is bound to have a major influence on how managers treat their personnel, on morale within the organization, on how indicators of program performance are defined and recorded; and on many other factors that influence day-to-day program management.

Information Systems and Evaluation

All organizations operate under requirements to report to outside bodies. All programs must produce information for their host organization. All programs need information to help deal with unexpected events. All programs should have information to take advantage of new funding opportunities or to gain publicity. The better one's information and evaluation systems, the better one can meet these challenges. But those systems are difficult to implement and run. They require people to operate them, office support, a staff willing to accept the operation of those systems, and, in this day and age, a computer system.

In human, organizational, and monetary terms, the costs of information and evaluation systems increase as programs mature. The systems are least expensive and most effective when instituted prior to the start of service delivery. Anyone who doubts this assertion need only ponder the answer to two questions. How easy is it to get people to use new forms or to revamp existing record-keeping policies? How useful is it for an evaluator to have intimate first-hand knowledge of a program's beginnings and the course of its program's development?

The best information and evaluation systems are built into a program from its beginning. In that way one can budget the necessary resources, structure good data collection, and foster organizational norms that are conducive to the smooth operation of information collection and evaluation.

THE UNIQUE NATURE OF PREVENTION PROGRAMS IN MENTAL HEALTH

All prevention programs have three unique characteristics that set them apart from most other types of programs: mass targeting, imprecise timing of treatment administration, and extended time frames. *Mass targeting* is necessary because the nature of prevention implies dealing with people who have not yet manifested a problem. No matter how good one's ability to determine a high risk population, a relatively high proportion of one's clientele will not need one's service. Indicators of risk are necessarily imprecise and false negatives are inevitable. *Timing of treatment:* assuming that a person will manifest a problem, when is the most auspicious time to prevent the problem's onset? More important, are there times when prevention efforts will have no effects at all, or have negative effects? Few prevention settings—especially in mental health—can answer these questions with any degree of certainty. *Extended time frames:* prevention programs by their nature have relatively long time periods between the application of a treatment and the ability to observe the effect of the treatment. After all, few prevention efforts focus on problems that would become immediately apparent absent an intervention.

In addition to these aspects of all prevention efforts, there are added difficulties for the case of mental health. First, the notion of attempting prevention is not as generally accepted as it is with other types of health programs. Second, there is less faith in the idea that once attempted, prevention efforts in mental health can have worthwhile consequences. Third, any data brought to support the efficacy of prevention in mental health will rely on the social and behavioral sciences—branches of science that lack credibility in many people's eyes. Finally, except for dramatic situations such as suicide, heavy substance abuse, or homelessness, it is difficult to make a convincing case that mental health issues represent serious public health or social welfare problems.

Thus problems with planning prevention programs in mental health can be conceptualized as a matrix, as seen in Table 1.1.

I hope to demonstrate in the remainder of this chapter that each of these characteristics poses special problems for the effective planning of prevention programs in mental health. Although I will not cover each cell of the matrix in detail, I hope to bring enough examples to demonstrate how this structure can be used to anticipate problems that may arise.

TABLE 1.1   Structure for Identifying Difficulties in Planning Prevention
            Programs in Mental Health

	Mass targeting	Timing of intervention	Extended time frames	Reputation of M.H.
Need analysis				
Program justification				
Consensus building				
Information and evaluation systems				

ILLUSTRATIVE EXAMPLES

Mass Targeting

Estimates of need tend to be inflated because they are based on imprecise "risk" factors, and because the apparent low cost of prevention (compared to treatment) encourages broad definitions of who should be served. Thus many more people will be identified as needing a prevention service than could truly benefit from it. The tendency to mass target a prevention program introduces uncertainties that make it difficult to estimate who—or how many—should be served. Even if the cost of service is of little consequence, these ambiguities still make it difficult to plan outreach programs, determine requirements for staff, or choose among different means of service delivery.

There are blessed occasions when the cost of service delivery is so low, when the delivery of service is so easy, and when the potential value is so high, that careful calculations involving target populations are unnecessary. A good example comes from our chapter on gerontology, where people who normally circulate in a community are asked to keep an eye out for elderly residents who may be in trouble. It costs little, for example, to ask postal workers to check on cases where an elderly person's mail suddenly lies uncollected. Opportunities for these high payoff, minimal cost possibilities must be sought, but we cannot define the limits of prevention programming by those opportunities.

The imprecision mentioned above extends to difficulties with program justification. No matter what the language of that justification—dollars, quality of life, or anything else—some estimate of amount of gain is necessary. As imprecision in estimates of need increases, estimates of gains from the program become more problematical.

Finally, consider the impact that imprecision will have on evaluation. The evaluator's assumption has to be that everyone who receives a treatment may in fact be affected by that treatment. Outcome data from people who cannot be helped are averaged with data from people who can be helped. As a result, empirical estimates of treatment effectiveness will inevitably decrease.

The more highly charged a political environment, the greater will be these difficulties. Consider what is needed to establish federal funding for prevention. First, there must be a "policy climate" that is conducive to the idea of prevention. Second, there must be specific beliefs that prevention in mental health is a better investment than any number of other mental health programs. How easy will it be to maintain such beliefs absent evaluation data that are perceived as valid, and that are cast in terms of politically relevant payoffs? How easy will it be to generate such data, given an evaluation context that must of necessity yield relatively weak estimates of success? It is because planners must have a keen appreciation of such difficulties that we have included a chapter on federal perspectives on prevention programming in mental health.

Timing of Treatment Administration

A critical aspect of planning is ensuring that appropriate treatments are delivered at the most auspicious times. Uncertainties about appropriate timing for prevention efforts in mental health can make it extremely difficult to build a consensus as to what constitutes an effective service that is worth providing.

As an example, consider the problems involved in school consultation, as discussed in another of this book's chapters. There is tremendous competition for students' time in a school system. Cognitive skills, physical education, cultural activities; proponents of these and many other topics are constantly vying for allocations of time during the school day. To succeed in that competition, proponents of prevention must start with a clear idea of when their activities will be most effective, and how much programming they should demand at various times in children's school careers.

Extended Time Frames

The long delay between treatment administration and the possible onset of a problem can cause difficulties in building a consensus to institute a program. As resources become scarce these difficulties are likely to increase. This is because the scarcer the resources, the greater the tendency to commit funds to immediate problems. It is not easy to argue that present difficulties should be slighted in favor of preventing problems that, if they occur at all, will affect later generations of politicians, policymakers, and health care professionals. This problem is reflected in our chapter on community mental health, a system that is fighting for survival. Community mental health services are being determined more and more by what is directly reimbursable. In most cases that means direct service for immediately apparent conditions. Thus supporters of prevention will have to work even harder against strong economic forces that are making it more and more difficult to justify service for problems that are not yet manifest.

Another set of problems is posed for evaluators who must deal with the long times between treatment and observation of its effects. If nothing else, powerful evaluation of prevention programs require all of the considerable funding, logistic support, and methodological rigor of longitudinal research designs. In addition, evaluators are faced with the added requirements of conceptualizing and measuring intermediate treatment goals.

This is because program managers and funders will need some guidance before any long-term effectiveness data can be accumulated. Both information systems and evaluation efforts must be adequate for these additional data requirements.

Special Characteristics of
Prevention in Mental Health

It is particularly difficult to justify mental health prevention because of the frequently encountered demand to frame the justification in terms of dollars, or in terms of some other widely recognized, easily defined "social good." Very often the justification for a mental health prevention program must be cast in terms of "quality of life," or "social competency," or similar terms that are not as cogent as money, or employment rates, or reading achievement. No matter how sympathetic a policymaker may be to a prevention program, political constraints often force one to opt for the most tangible benefits that can be achieved. If there must be a choice between a program to increase children's reading skills or a program to increase their interpersonal problem-solving ability, smart money will ride on the reading program. These difficulties are illustrated by our chapter on self-help. Why should such groups be supported? Because they are a worthwhile resource that improve participants' quality of life? Because they can reduce the need for costly clinical interventions? Because they can potentiate the impact of clinical interventions? All three reasons appear to have some legitimacy, but those that offer the most tangible outcomes are often the hardest to prove; self-help groups (particularly the anonymous groups) often are reluctant to engage in formal evaluation studies.

In writing this chapter I do not mean to imply that good planning for prevention in mental health is a lost cause. As the chapters in this book will show so well, good prevention planning can be done. It is being done now. But as planners of prevention programs in mental health, we face special challenges that must be met with deliberation, determination, and creativity. I hope that by articulating the structure of these problems, I have provided a sense of where difficulties are likely to arise, and how they may be overcome. As you read the remaining chapters, you will see the techniques others have used to meet these challenges.

Reference

Morell, J. A. (1981). Evaluation of prevention: Implications from a general model. *Prevention in the human services* (Vol. 1). New York: Haworth.

Chapter 2

PREVENTION PLANNING AS SOCIAL AND ORGANIZATIONAL CHANGE

MARSHALL SWIFT and THOMAS W. WEIRICH

This chapter describes the creation and use of a working model for the planning of prevention programs in mental health. The model is based upon the fundamental processes of social and organizational change. It is intended to facilitate planning efforts by providing a framework for bringing together concept, reality, and research. The model has evolved over a number of years, emerging from the interaction of practical experience, trial and error, success and failure, and a growing body of useful theoretical and empirical literature. The present model also reflects the contributions of many practitioners who have actually used its ideas in the planning and delivery of real-world prevention programs. Theirs is perhaps the sternnest test. We hope and expect that the model will continue to evolve as it is used and criticized. It is intended to be a living, working tool, justified only by its continued meaning and utility.

BACKGROUND

Our belief that an overall framework for planning is needed is based upon experience in developing prevention programs for people of all ages, for a variety of ethnic and socioeconomic groups, and in a wide range of community mental health settings. Most of this occurred in a center dominated by the traditional mental illness treatment approach, but accepting prevention as one of the center's components. Although legitimate, prevention was conceived of and even assumed to be provided through existing clinical outreach services. However, perhaps because of our affiliation with an academic, research-oriented institution and our beliefs in analysis and investigation, we questioned these traditional assumptions.

Our analysis of the initial prevention efforts led us to the firm conclusion that the goals and methods for prevention were different from the models guiding traditional mental health treatment processes. Indeed, the foundation values and ideas that made prevention meaningful were radically different from the traditional paradigm. More recently, Cowen (1982) affirmed our earlier conclusion when he described "trail blazing program paradigms in primary prevention," which were published in a recent *Journal of Community Psychology, Prevention Edition*. Cowen noted that although the nine program models accepted for publication were widely diverse, they were substantially as well as conceptually dissimilar from orthodox mental health programs. Their content and supporting knowledge bases extend across diverse domains both within psychology (developmental, educational, organization, environmental, social) and well beyond it.

The differences were not only procedural, nor just tactical. There were fundamental differences in the central ideas that made prevention meaningful and in the central processes that made prevention a dynamic enterprise. The most essential differences were the number and variety of people (actors, stakeholders, constituents) involved in planning, implementation, and assessment, and the dynamic nature of the development process itself. In addition, it was clear that there were tremendous pressures on prevention to prove itself "scientifically" even in its infancy. Thus traditional program planning and implementation models were inappropriate for prevention, and a more suitable guide was needed. Fortunately, developments in the organizational planning literature were a good match with our growing body of practical wisdom (see Van de Ven & Koenig, 1976).

AIMS AND OBJECTIVES

The overall aim of our framework is to provide a guide and a set of principles that will be useful to planners, practitioners, and researchers in the planning, implementation, and evaluation of successful prevention programs. The framework is based upon the processes of psychosocial and organizational change that underlie planned change and knowledge application. Three objectives provide the focus:

(1) to provide a basis for recognizing the wide variety of *stakeholders and constituencies* important to prevention programs and to guide their effective inclusion in planning, implementation, and evaluation;
(2) to identify and give direction to the basic *planning elements and change processes* that are involved in prevention planning, implementation, and evaluation; and
(3) to promote the *integration of applied research* into planning, implementation, and assessment of prevention programs.

Each of these objectives will be discussed in turn.

STAKEHOLDERS AND CONSTITUENCIES

We sometimes forget that the planning and implementation of prevention programs is essentially a social process. There will be many different kinds of people involved in a variety of social interactions. Good planning anticipates who the participants will be and attempts to guide their activities. Of course, some people will become program clients, whereas others will hold basic staff roles. Many planners make the mistake of stopping there, though the list of relevant participants extends much farther. Any individual, group, organization, or social entity capable of taking meaningful action in relation to the prevention program should be considered and encouraged to become a significant *actor*. This point has not always been so obvious. In earlier prevention projects prior to emphasis upon the idea, we found that teachers involved in a program were, at best, only tolerant of the preventive interventions, and at times were even hostile. They objected, "I don't think it's a good idea to miss class," or "The children's behavior is worse after the stimulation of the program." It is not surprising that teacher behavior did not change from reactive to proactive as hoped. Furthermore, few school administrators had any significant knowledge of, or commitment to, the intervention program. We believed that program failures were not because of the inadequacy of the particular intervention used, but instead were due to the failure of the overall implementation plan and approach. An NIMH report (1973, p. 5) came to a similar conclusion:

> The first important point related to the success or failure of a mental health consultation program is that success may bear little relationship to the qualifications of the staff of the Community Mental Health Center providing the services. In fact, they may be of the highest calibre, expertly trained and dedicated, but be denied the opportunity to provide the very services the school district indicates it desperately needs. The underlying basis for this problem often is *the inability of mental health specialists to understand the internal dynamics of* the school system—the moral dilemmas educators face on a daily basis, the political pressures with which they must constantly deal, the conflicts among staff related to differences in educational philosophy, and the conflicting demands and pressures from parents and state education codes. In short, *failure to understand the social dynamics* of the schools (a subject not usually included in the curriculum of training programs for mental health professionals) *often is the single most significant determinant of success or failure.* (emphasis added)

The NIMH report emphasized the folly of focusing too narrowly on the prevention clients while ignoring the many other actors who have an interest in a program. Of course a more comprehensive viewpoint increases the complexity of the situation. This difficulty can be managed by categorizing the important actors into levels, ranging from those most immediately involved in the program—the target group and beneficiaries—through those with more limited involvement—such as gatekeepers and referral agents—to the general yet relevant environment of policymakers. Our model (see Figure 2.1) explicitly recognizes these many other levels and provides for their meaningful inclusion in planning.

The use of intervention levels gives the situation more form and structure, but lacks the substance and content needed to make the actors real and meaningful. This is accomplished by articulating each actor's perspective or point of view on the program. Is the actor positive, neutral, or negative about prevention? Does he or she have strong feelings about it? How does the idea of intervention prior to evidence of pathology fit into the actor's values and interests? How important or salient is prevention? These are the types of questions that must be answered to understand what stake the actor has in prevention, and thus to understand how the actor will behave in relation to the program.

It quickly becomes apparent that there will be a great diversity of perspectives and needs, and thus a great diversity of expectations for each program. This translates into diverse and often conflicting program success criteria. Recipients, for example, clearly expect effective solutions to problems and concrete benefits. Funders, on the other hand, want program efficiency and accountability. The scientific community will be more concerned with the validity of the program's knowledge base and the quality of supporting research evidence.

Given this diversity, communication among involved actors is an essential process, but unfortunately it is frequently a serious problem. Our model seeks to facilitate effective communication by providing a common language, a set of ideas and terms, and even a graphic representation of the program for planners and other participants to share. By listing and defining essential program elements, including basic assumptions and ideas, and connecting these to each actor's special point of view, the model

Planning Elements	Individual (A)	Caregivers (B)	Organizations (C)	Networks (D)	Community (E)	Policy (F)
			Levels of Interaction and Change			
(1) People • Targets/beneficiaries • Stakeholders • Constituencies	(1.A)					(1.F)
(2) Ideas • Goals/objectives • Ideals/values • Knowledge base		(2.B)			(2.E)	
(3) Performance • Impacts by types • Criteria			(3.C)	(3.D)		
(4) Action • Tasks • Methods • Tactics			(4.C)	(4.D)		
(5) Resources • Programmatic • Strategic		(5.B)			(5.E)	
(6) Politics • Policy/strategy • Power	(6.A)					(6.F)

Figure 2.1 A Framework for Prevention Planning

supplies a cell-by-cell picture of who will be involved, what goals and tasks are to be achieved, and how and where an intervention is to occur. The model also allows for the consideration and questioning of why an element is included in a plan.

Finally, the model provides real benefits beyond communication. It supplies a shared framework for critical decision making and promotes needed collaboration among the many actors. It guides each of them to focus on the critical aspects of a program at each development step, while allowing for the inevitable differences among perspectives. Points of agreement can be identified and made explicit. Perhaps more important, differences can be clarified and examined within a meaningful context. Underlying assumptions and rationales, interests, and values can be articulated. Thus the framework serves both to define and solidify the bonds between collaborators and to bridge the gaps between differing perspectives. Successful change requires the formation of solid partnerships, strong alliances, and effective coalitions, and the model is a tool to this end.

PLANNING ELEMENTS AND CHANGE PROCESSES

A successful prevention plan is an effective combination of a number of ingredients. We call these ingredients *planning elements*. They are the components of change, the pieces that must be carefully and strategically analyzed, matched, and brought together, and then managed throughout the change process. The model provides the planner with a means of identifying the most important individual elements, and with a framework for thinking about the total scope of the program in an integrated and holistic manner. This "big picture" approach makes the diversity of the particular elements and activities in any program more comprehensible and reduces the extreme complexity that develops to manageable proportions. Most important, the model provides a framework for programmatic decision making.

The model identifies six categories of planning elements: people, ideas, performance, action, resources, and politics (see Figure 2.1). We will briefly define and discuss each category here, saving detailed analysis for a later section. The first planning element is *people*. Prevention planning is a social process aimed at supporting a social-psychological service, and thus people are a fundamental concern. As we have stated earlier, it is useful to think of the social dimension in levels. It is also useful to distinguish among target groups and beneficiaries, stakeholders, and general constituencies.

Prevention planning is also a cultural process and *ideas* are the second planning element. This component includes normative ideas such as goals and objectives, values and ideals, and more cognitive and descriptive ideas such as those in theoretical and research bases.

Because prevention is an applied, achievement-oriented endeavor, *performance* is an essential element. It is important to specify the concrete impacts that are expected in terms of attitudes, knowledge, and behavior. Measurable criteria for monitoring and judging program activities should also be established.

The conversion of the prevention plan into a reality of course requires real and effective *action*. The plan should integrate action with the tactical context and specify the general methods to be used, as well as specific tasks to be done. The action component provides the means necessary to achieve the ends articulated in the ideas component.

No plan can be accomplished without money, facilities, information, staff, and other essential *resources*. Some resources will be needed for actual program tasks and work. But the plan should also include sufficient resources for the administrative, planning, and policy activities.

The final planning element is *politics,* a recognition that all social and organizational change involves political, power-based activity. Rather than neglecting or ignoring this dimension, our model makes politics an explicit and important component of change.

No prevention program bursts into the world fully developed and operational. There is a long process of development, growth, and maturation. The metaphor of the "life cycle of change" is a useful conceptual aid for appreciating the dynamics of this process. The life of a prevention program can be divided into stages and steps, each with its own distinctive set of problems and requirements (see Brager & Holloway, 1978; Van de Ven, 1980). The planning and work involved during early initiation of a program, for example, are very different from the requirements during mature program operation. Sensitivity to such stages of development is crucial to effective planning.

Program stages are important because different combinations of planning elements are appropriate and most effective at different times and in different circumstances. Accurately defining the situation and then finding the right combination of planning ingredients, what Van de Ven (1980) calls "strategic matching," is the key to successful prevention planning. Our model provides a framework for this continuing process of program reconstruction.

RESEARCH INTEGRATION

Prevention has suffered from the peculiar pressures of being expected to prove itself even before having established and perfected field programs. It has not enjoyed the support to enable the development of a research base for respected services to provide credible evidence of success. Thus the "scientific mandate," the demand for evidence, has been problematic. Practitioners typically are not skilled at research, and it has been difficult to build a knowledge and research base. The need for a guide to the integration of research in prevention planning became evident following an analysis of data from some early prevention efforts in our community mental health center (Swift, 1976a, 1976b) and from an NIMH national study (1973) of similar activities. These studies revealed that the focus of "prevention" activities was almost always upon a small group with little attempt made to generalize to other populations, or even to others within similar populations. The process most often involved removing at-risk participants (usually children in school) from a classroom setting for a special program. The program goal was to prevent the need for psychotherapeutic intervention. Neither our research group nor the NIMH research team could find any impact upon the behavior of similar other populations at risk in the same setting, nor could differences between those receiving the program and their peers be identified at the end of a program.

The lack of adequate sampling designs and comparison groups made generalization of findings impossible. The lack of detailed program descriptions made transferability of program components extremely difficult. Most important, the lack of elementary measurement and resultant evidence made the credibility of any claims very low. Thus any argument, political or scientific, was too often (but not totally) limited to appeals to intuition and emotion.

Programs designed with our guide are more amenable to the scientific mandate and experimentation because the generation of meaningful data is built into program design. Within the general thrust of a program, a variety of specific techniques can be tested and compared to determine which prevention methods are most effective. The operating program becomes, in effect, its own experimental station, constantly assessing and reassessing the merit of program alternatives. Thus the possibility of program generalizations and transfer becomes enhanced.

PRINCIPLES

The objective for this section is to present some general action principles that we have developed as guides to the successful implementation of prevention programs. Although such guides are helpful, we know that each setting and each effort are unique (Nadler, 1981a, 1981b), and there is no single, universal blueprint. General principles must be carefully adapted to each situation and should not be pursued ritualistically. Nevertheless, the change literature and our early experiences convinced us that guiding principles and a model for action improve planning and implementation efforts. Further, we believe that they can ultimately help achieve real changes in preventive mental health services.

One of our first and most valuable realizations was that we needed to identify allies and search for resources beyond the boundaries of the mental health system. It is not possible to mount the kind of prevention programs needed without coalitions of outside supporters, agreements among organizations, and inputs of outside resources. On an even more subtle level, successful prevention programs require changes in the thinking of influential people outside of the program itself. In 1972 Glasscote et al. concluded,

> The magnitude of trying to provide an optimum opportunity for every child to develop to his greatest potential is far too great to be accomplished by such small facilities as mental health services. Such services are in a good position to develop principles and techniques that might be widely applied, but perhaps the most promising approaches lie in the area of providing family-life education to young people, through the schools, and to increasing the information, competence, and comfort of people whose work involved children. (Glasscote, Fishman & Sonis, 1972, p. 34)

The concept of widely applying principles and techniques to those outside of the mental health system was credible and compatible with our proactive view of making prevention available to the general population. The idea of working with others in collaborative ways, and of working through others by enhancing their own skills, became hallmarks of our approach. Thus our first principle is as follows.

> I. Define the *people* relevant to a prevention program's goals broadly across a number of social levels, including target groups, direct beneficiaries, and other *stakeholders*.

Important illustrations of stakeholders are the many disciplines and caregivers that come in contact with at risk target groups (e.g., the frail elderly, children of the mentally ill). How can programs involve multiple professions and their skills in an effective prevention effort? In the social work literature Litwak (1971) suggested the establishment of "balanced partnerships" between personnel in different fields and agencies and between agencies and the citizens they serve for the ultimate benefit of the clientele. Van de Ven (1980) used the term "rolling alliances" to describe the continuous process of joining together diverse interests in goal-directed but temporary coalitions. Our experience confirmed that for a prevention program to be accepted, implemented, and sustained, understanding and collaboration among agencies and citizens were essential. Prevention programs are best achieved, not as packaged procedures superimposed by mental health professionals but as partnerships among many stakeholders, professionals as well as lay people.

At a more general level, the process is also one of building a *constituency* for prevention. Perhaps more so than many other social problems, prevention requires an elaborate campaign to generate political support (see Tallman, 1976). Prevention experts have observed,

> Despite its logical attractiveness, there is little in the way of an existing constituency demanding primary prevention compared to that which exists for programs of treatment or rehabilitation. . . . Health and peace have in common the fact that it is difficult to organize a constituency that defines its need as the maintenance of a positive state of affairs. (Broskowski & Baker, 1974, pp. 709, 716).

We believe that building a viable constituency requires involvement of potential consumers or their representatives. Typically this has been interpreted to mean holding meetings with various members of a community to explain a program, to obtain information, and/or to organize general support. Commonly, no strategic plan or set of performance objectives is used. Our experience has been that this is not enough. For example, in one of our early unsuccessful efforts in a school setting, the school principal was very rarely part of the planning and ongoing implementation and evaluation processes. However, we learned that the school administrator in a large urban system is "at risk" when innovations occur in his or her school, and thus has a significant "stake" in new programs. We learned that we also had to consider the organizational leader, the teachers, and other caregivers in the prevention setting to function more effectively, handle emotional difficulties, and thus receive benefits from the program. When their interests are addressed, they are more willing to collaborate on programs for the children. Thus our second principle is as follows:

II. Manage the *politics* of a prevention effort by increasing cooperation and collaboration among the many actors involved. Form *partnerships,* create *alliances,* build *coalitions, and generate a constituency* for prevention.

A second realization that emerged from our earliest investigations was that we had to define *our own* ideas and approaches more carefully before we could effectively communicate and share them with others. A wide variety of people were involved and thus had to understand what we were attempting and why. Their acceptance of our basic ideas was a foundation for their involvement. The first step was clarifying what we meant by prevention.

In 1967, Caplan and Grunebaum introduced the idea that prevention was the "reduction of mental illness, as well as to promote mental health," giving a very broad base to the term. Klein and Goldston (1976) later asserted, "The use of the word prevention should be limited to primary prevention. To refer to early treatment as secondary or rehabilitation activities as tertiary prevention contributes to the confusion and diminishes the usefulness of the term. . . . Prevention is directed toward reducing the incidence of a highly predictable undesirable consequence." As it evolved this definition now includes the promotion of mental health. Thus, for example, one goal might be to prevent disruptive or maladaptive behavior in the classroom, and a second to promote productive interpersonal behavior to facilitate emotional development. Subsequently, Goldston (1977) noted that the basic principles and practices of primary prevention emerge out of our commonly shared ideology about community mental health, including the following:

(1) A commitment to increasing the mental health of the entire community, not just to treatment of the psychiatric casualties.

(2) A serious effort to involve community institutions "accompanied by an awareness that the mental health enterprise is but one among many help-giving agencies concerned with the mental health of the population."

(3) Public health concepts and practices, because "(a) no condition has been controlled or prevented merely by treating victims. Community based programs before-the-fact (vs. early diagnosis and treatment) are needed to prevent problems; and (b) a key question is 'how well' is the community? Rather than 'how sick'"

Our thinking was further influenced by Hollister (1976) from the psychiatric perspective, who emphasized a less grand first step in identifying the object of prevention. The first issue he advised was that preventionists must be clear about what we can prove:

> Humanity is the keynote in setting the goals of prevention programs. Some day, we hope we shall learn how to prevent the major psychoses, neuroses and the character disorders, but until that day we must settle for more humble objectives. Those of us in psychological fields can wisely borrow from the experience gained in preventing physical disorders. Even in physical medicine the first prevention efforts were not to prevent serious disease processes like heart disease, cancer or arthritis. Their first efforts were to prevent injuries, hemorrages, debilitation from fever, wound infections and disabilities. Instead of rejecting prevention in the mental health field because we cannot yet for sure prevent schizophrenia, let us, like physical medicine has done, start humbly with today's knowledge and gain experience step-by-step. (Hollister, 1976, p. 1)

To become more precise in our thinking about the definition of prevention and about the steps we were prepared to take, we started with the premise that the goal for prevention is to decrease the likelihood that individuals will develop emotional-behavioral difficulties, and to accomplish this interventions must be made "before-the-fact" rather than after problems occur. Applying our first principle, our access to the individual was to be through others on a number of different levels, by bringing them knowledge of how to prevent problems and how to reach large numbers of people simultaneously. Our third principle is as follows:

> III. The *idea* of prevention, in terms of both its ideals and goals, and its approaches and methods, must be carefully articulated, shared, managed, and promoted throughout the planning and implemenation process.

Prevention is caught between conflicting pressures for action and for research. We have described the absence of a research orientation in many prevention programs, and the resultant lack of evidence on program consequences. Contemporary circumstances do not allow the comfort of low visibility and generous support, but neither is there enough time or resources to mount a giant research effort. The need is for an integration of existing and accruing research with ongoing planning and action at the local level. To be viable, this integration must produce meaningful evidence for general audiences and useful information for local stakeholders. We think such an integration is possible (see Hermalin & Weirich, 1982; Weirich & Hermalin, 1982), and can serve both general and local interests.

To fit with the other general planning principles, the research effort should be highly participatory and collaborative among all of the parties involved in the prevention program. The aim is to establish a "community of inquiry" around prevention. This community is a loose coalition of actors and interests that share a commitment to prevention, but who are willing to continuously seek greater understanding of it and more effective programs. Through constant questioning, evaluation, and revision, they will keep the idea of prevention alive, while improving concrete programs. The research process is shared, ongoing, and "alive," not a single formalized study by an academic. The bottom line for this group is local utility, and they will have a very practical orientation to research. Data collection, analysis, and utilization will be tied to specific program issues and needs. Specific efforts will vary in style in each planning stage. The process is facilitated by clear specifications of action plans and tasks, and careful articulation of performance expectations and criteria. Because these are essential components of well-managed programs, the research dimension need not place an unreasonable burden on prevention practice. The benefits will justify the effort. Thus, our last action principle is as follows:

> IV. An applied research process should be an integral part of prevention planning and implementation. Research should be a meaningful and useful component of each stage of prevention development.

THE MODEL

The model presented in Figure 2.1 represents in graphic form the concepts, assumptions, and principles we have discussed. Across the top of the table the model first identifies six levels of action and change: individual, caregivers, organizations, networks, community, and policy. The content of each level is located in the respective columns. Second, the six planning elements are listed vertically to form the rows. The categories are people, ideas, performance, action, resources, and politics. The combination of levels and elements is a 6 × 6 property space, containing 36 cells. Each cell represents the information needed to specify each planning element at each level of action. The content of the cells will describe different planning issues, different information needs, and different implications for action and research.

The general thinking process moves from a general identification of constituencies and targets at each level through increasingly specific articulation of ideas, performance expectations, and actions. Thinking then begins to become more generalized, as resource needs are spelled out for the program and for strategic action. Finally, returning to a more generalized realm, planning and program politics are considered. The application of the model forces one to follow this hourglass-like thinking scheme, focusing then refocusing attention.

The best way to describe the model is through a concrete illustration of its use in our own prevention efforts. Before doing so, it must be noted that although most of the examples focus upon children, in practice the model can and has been applied to specific prevention programs across the age span as well as for statewide planning (Hall, 1983). Child-directed examples come most readily to mind because we are reporting upon our work. However, as Lorion (1984), reporting upon a national prevention survey carried out by the Community Division of the American Psychological Association, noted, "Survey responses indicated that prevention/promotion efforts address a very wide range of target problems.... Not surprisingly, nearly one-half (of 265 projects reviewed) identified children and/or adolescents as their primary target." Nevertheless, adults (17%) and age groups combined (27%) as well as the elderly (5%) also were targets of preventive interventions. It is our contention that these programs would be enhanced in process, outcome, and survivability through the use of the prevention program model described in this article.

AN ILLUSTRATION OF THE MODEL

Individuals

The ultimate beneficiary of prevention activities is the individual. We intend to improve the individual's life and well-being and to promote positive growth. But prevention does not view the individual in isolation, treating each case as unique. Prevention planning considers groups or categories of individuals in similar life circumstances. These circumstances may be normal developmental stages where progress is essential to immediate and long-term well-being, or they may be life experiences high in stress, or a combination of developmental and stress factors that cause specialized needs. For example, developmental issues include home to school transitions or retirement; stressful events could include death, divorce, or unemployment; and combination events are illustrated by teenage pregnancy. Forquer (1981/1982, p. 10) has written,

> The life span of every human being is characterized by a series of progressive, predictable developmental stages. In each of these stages skills are expected to emerge or be developed which can eventuate in the adequate preparation of the individual for adequate functioning. In order for this psychological development to occur, certain environmental conditions need to exist. The goal of primary prevention activities is to decrease the occurrence of mental disorder to promoting healthy coping behavior and enhancing the competency of vulnerable and normal populations.

We designate these categories of people as "at-risk groups," and make them the targets of prevention efforts. Ideals and goals are formulated to guide activities. Our aims are to decrease the incidence of problems among at-risk populations and/or to promote the competence of at-risk individuals to manage normal and specific stressful conditions successfully.

Following our first principle, however, we must realize that there are other potential beneficiaries who have a stake in the prevention effort. Frequently, these others can become an essential part of the program.

For example, several years ago we created a program for children in an at-risk population of preschoolers to decrease the incidence of maladaptive functioning in kindergarten. Our earlier research (a longitudinal study of similar children begun in 1968) had documented the frequency and nature of maladaptive behavior in kindergarten, and its relation to third grade failure and behavioral problems (Spivack & Swift, 1977). From the perspective of the in-the-classroom behavior of the children the program was successful.

There was, however, some disquiet and personal unhappiness expressed by some of the parents. We knew that the lack of appropriate skills among many lower-class mothers was itself a reason for the need for early school programs for the children. Although parent involvement, motivation, and enthusiasm are very important assets to enhancing the child's interest and involvement, these attributes alone do not change the fact that many lower-class mothers remain unable to involve themselves in even the most rudimentary preparation for their child's effective development (Swift, 1970). In short, although the concept of parent involvement is emphasized by almost all programs for preschool children, there is little evidence of specifically tailored parent-focused programs—programs designed to promote the mental health of lower-class parents as one integrated aspect of a preventive intervention with their children.

Most middle-class mental health oriented parent education programs are educational or cognitive processes designed to help parents gain a better understanding of their children through knowledge building. To some degree, it appears this model has been retained for use with the lower-class parent. However, insight and information are of little value without adequate development of concrete communication skills for the parents themselves—skills that evidence indicates relate to the mental health of the adults as well as their children (Chilman, 1966). Chilman noted that the nature of the communication process used by the lower-class parents like those with whom we were working militated against the use of discussion and information sharing for problem solving. Furthermore, our experience with this population indicated they did not regularly attend meetings or join groups, particularly when the purpose of the group was only "to hold discussions."

These findings suggested that the mothers need activities designed specifically to increase their confidence and ability to affect the growth and learning of their children in an immediately valued manner (i.e., their own self-esteem). In creating such a program, the unique characteristics of the mother attempting to raise children in an atmosphere of poverty had to be taken into consideration. The poverty mother frequently needs a great deal of support and nurturing herself. The loneliness and social isolation of many of the mothers suggested the use of group activities. It was emphasized that these groups focus upon ways in which the mothers themselves, working in a group, could have maximum oppportunities for quick success in meaningful skill development. Thus though we began with an intervention designed to enhance children's interpersonal problem-solving skills so that maladaptive behaviors in preschool and kindergarten would be prevented, a new goal to enhance the parents' view of their role in the development of their children, as well as increase positive feelings about themselves in the process, was added. We now had two target groups, two sets of goals, and parents as stakeholders, and we needed an approach that could address these issues simultaneously.

The children not only needed to increase attentiveness to school tasks (i.e., pay attention when the teacher talked, read stories, and so on) but they also needed mothers who could confidently reinforce the teacher's actions (e.g., using books for stories) in ways that were valued by mother and child.

To accomplish this, we needed a methodology to increase parenting skills for socially, intellectually, and educationally limited parents. We knew that a number of variables distinguished the communication style of the lower-class mother and her child and that these styles were related to various types of child behavior such as acting out, hyperactivity, hyper-aggressivity, temper tantrums, poor frustration tolerance, and other manifestations of tension (Chilman, 1966).

The intervention approach that involved both target groups was the use of preschool books as the method of communication skill development to enhance the mother's verbal skills.

Caregivers

It has been our experience that such a program of direct intervention by mental health professionals no matter how successful is not the most effective or cost efficient prevention approach. If a prevention program is to be successful and lasting, consideration and planning for the significant engagement of diverse intervention levels must be developed from inception. The most immediate level is the caregivers.

Caregivers are those who provide individuals with beneficial or potentially beneficial interactions in a variety of settings such as schools and public or private agencies: teachers, principals, clergy, coaches, police-community liaison officers, and social caseworkers are examples. Although outside of the direct mental health delivery system, their potential contribution to the prevention of mental health problems is significant. In the natural course of their work they are confronted with opportunities to promote mental health every day. All too often, however, they are ill-prepared to respond to the mental health needs presented, or they feel conflicts between the task to be accomplished and the needs of the person involved: The police officer must ascertain the facts from the rape victim, the teacher must increase reading skills.

And yet, even when caregivers are skilled at meeting both their job tasks and the emotional needs of their clients, they are still often caught in a dilemma. It appears to the caregiver that their organization and its management have other agendas—agendas that impede or actually forbid the caregiver from responding to the emotional needs of their clients. We have learned that too many caregivers working in today's organizations are themselves under great stress due to feelings of powerlessness, overwhelming work demands, conflicting and frequently changing instructions, and job insecurity. In our approach these stressors upon those at the caregiver level are considered when we plan and implement mental health prevention programs. Once again this is another reason (in addition to building stakeholders) why our model is designed to plan for and handle the needs of people at various levels.

Continuing our earlier illustration, the use of preschool books for children and parents led us to involve the community services department of the public library. A specialist in children's work was needed to help create techniques and to carry out the project. No special skills were proposed for the librarian, beyond understanding the mental health implications of the project. The library staff had to begin this work with the skills they already had, and we had to reassure them that they had the basic skills needed. It was made clear that the Mental Health Center staff would be responsible for handling the concerns of the librarians, programming difficulties, and administrative issues. A formalized agreement for a ten-week exploratory program was made. Over time the librarian became very skilled at working with functionally illiterate parents, and even continued to use the new skills after the program. Other librarians were trained by the original one, giving the library a new skilled resource for community service. The parents and children involved benefited from other health services and their growing competencies in story telling and communication.

Once trained the more successful mothers were involved in recruiting and training a cadre of new mothers for the next school year.

Organizations

To an ever-increasing degree, organizations dominate modern society and influence our lives. This is no less true for prevention, and it must be built into prevention planning. Organizations are an important setting for prevention programs, and can even be the focus for a prevention effort. To work with organizations successfully, the preventionist must come to terms with the dynamics of the organization itself. Organizations are complex and changing. The needs for which many public agencies were formed have modified and grown. Schools, for example, no longer just educate; many now provide breakfast and lunch, administer health services, organize athletic activities, and serve as community meeting places. Schools are also expected to serve all children, regardless of handicap, emotional difficulty, or intellectual capacity. Furthermore, the school must provide a hospitable working environment for increasingly frustrated and militant employees. In the context of their own environments the same issues emerge for private businesses as well as public agencies.

Most of these conflicting forces meet at the level of the organizational leader, and frequently the stresses of the job are reflected in leadership strain. In one of our surveys (Johnson, Healey, & Swift, 1981), for example, half of 44 school administrators rated themselves "moderately to extremely burned out" due to intergroup problems. Furthermore despite physical health similar to the general population (see *In Pursuit of Wellness,* 1979), they were far less apt to report a good sense of psychological well-being. Only 18% indicated their sense of emotional stability to be excellent as compared to 51% of a comparable group in the same age range. Furthermore only 60% indicated that they felt able to do all they wanted to even though they were physically able to do so (compared to 80% of the controls). Work issues for these school administrators were particularly complex because of the "person-in-the-middle" role they played within the organization: between and among teachers, counselors, and other support staff (caregivers), parents and community residents (community), and the superintendent and other district-wide directors (policy levels), as well as with other organizations such as police, community mental health centers, and welfare agencies (networks).

The significance of the school administrator's role and the impact of his or her effectiveness upon the educational progress and emotional development of children justified a prevention program focused upon this level of the organization. The goal of the project was to enable administrators to define and meet their multiple commitments to those above and below them and thereby decrease feelings of burnout and helplessness. We attempted such a program with a "modest beginning" (using Hollister's notion of beginning small and gaining experience) by engaging school administrators who revealed themselves to be at-risk due to emotional distress on the job. From the general population of the school, 44 administrators participated in a program designed to focus upon preventing the impact of stress and distress. We considered input from other organizational levels, and awareness of differing methods of intergroup problem solving at these levels. A similar program for teachers (caregivers) could have been run simultaneously. A number of guidelines are available for such prevention programs. (These and other programs focusing upon organizational development or team building can be identified through a literature search.)

Organizational-level programs can be evaluated to assess the degree of indirect impact upon the attitudes, knowledge, and behavior of caregivers (in this case the teachers). The ultimate preventive impact could be assessed in terms of its effect upon the behaviors and emotional difficulties of the children (Individual Level).

Carrying this concept one step further, Felner, Ginter, and Primavera (1982) targeted the organizational level for change by reorganizing the school environment for youngsters facing the potentially negative effects of the crisis of transition from junior to senior high school. To do so they restructured the role of homeroom teachers (caregivers) and increased peer social supports (community). Such a method, if tied to a program for principals and teachers, becomes much more possible because of the support it is likely to earn from them. Furthermore, it could be evaluated for effectiveness in reducing negative effects of stress upon three levels simultaneously.

Networks

The network level of our model evolved as we attempted to convey our prevention mission to others in the community. Historically, working at this level has been one of the most difficult for mental health professionals. Poor understanding of others' approaches and mandates creates suspicion, differing goals cause disagreement, and scarce resources bring competition. Yet, cooperation and collaboration among providers can produce programs not possible acting alone. We sought ways to overcome suspicions and misperceptions, to learn more about others' goals and approaches, and to share resources. It has been our experience that agency personnel, industrial leaders, and community groups are willing to open their doors and discuss cooperation. When interests can be matched for mutual benefit, there is a tendency to join in collaborative efforts. There is then a willingness to provide ideas and participate in interagency communication, provide space, and/or allot time for consultation. Some will enter into exchange agreements for resources or facilities, or agree to mutual referral compacts. Research suggests that formalized agreements among social service organizations promotes at least case-level interaction among line workers (Weirich & Perlmutter 1977).

In our earlier example, the ties created among the prevention program within a mental health center, the schools, and the library illustrated a simple network. Each of the parties benefited from the exchange, and the children and parents received improved service. The model depicted in Figure 2.1 reminds the planner to define each planning element at the network level so that the formation and maintenance of the network itself becomes a prevention effort.

Community

Prevention has a very important cultural dimension, involving the diffusion of ideas through a community. Thus prevention planning should include an educational component, aimed at those outside of the formal service delivery system. The aim should be to raise general consciousness about needs, prevention approaches, and available services. The prevention philosophy differs from the popular medical worldview, and people will have much to learn about its concepts and methods. The designation of "at-risk" groups based upon conceptual and research evidence rather than problem symptoms, for example, will be new to many communities.

At another level, the promotion of the prevention idea is essential to the mobilization of political support for prevention programs. Prevention must develop a constituency that will seek and support prevention efforts. Indeed, the survival of the prevention movement may depend more upon the existence of a strong and influential constituency than the technical merits of specific programs.

Our experience has been that there is a potential constituency for prevention, and many potential recipients become active when resources are made known and accessible to them, and when prevention is clearly tied to their personal interests and well-being. For example, with very rare exception most mothers want their children to do well in school, get along with teachers and peers, and achieve. However, most programs in poverty communities are for the children alone and do not significantly engage the parents. This is especially true when the parent has not been a successful learner. While the child receives more and more assistance outside of the home, the mother has nowhere to learn the skills that allow her the opportunity to participate in the education of her child. In this area, as in too many aspects of her life, the poverty mother feels and often is powerless to affect positively her life or the lives of her children. Often the mother who realizes that she lacks the skills necessary to help her child learn and achieve life goals adopts the feeling that she is unnecessary. Ironically, as her child gains more outside assistance, the mother feels that she is less of an impact upon his or her development. This adds more frustration, increasing the sense of worthlessness and alienation.

However, when a program is designed to directly increase the useful skills of parents, they become prevention partners and advocates. Their interests and involvement can extend beyond the specific program to the promotion and support of prevention in general. One result of our involvement of parents, for example, was that the parents used their new skills to begin developing communication links with parents outside of the preschool. In this manner a local self-help movement developed.

In future projects we engaged some of the mothers who had "graduated" to train new program mothers. They used the books to engage other adults in the learning process, supporting and encouraging each other in turn. We discovered the grass-roots validity of self-help and made this one of our ultimate goals for the program. From this experience we demonstrated that community residents can and do aid the involvement of mental health specialists in their neighborhood. They provide information to neighbors, promote and support the appropriate use of prevention resources, and serve as peer teachers and role models and as an advocacy group.

Social Policy

Unfortunately most mental health personnel do not conceive of their role as including responsibility for influencing social policy. But, as community specialists we must be concerned with the policies and policymakers that affect all levels of the community. Very early in our experience, staff were challenged by a representative of an advisory committee to the mayor of Philadelphia to "demonstrate that you have a constituency for prevention." It was clear that we had planned no means of gathering evidence that people wanted prevention services or services beyond those provided for the mentally ill. Furthermore, in our community-based work we were constrained on a number of occasions by public policy that impeded or defeated implementation of a prevention program. For example, foster parents were forbidden by policy to develop a close attachment to foster infants, an attachment crucial to future emotional development; teenage girls could not receive sex education until they became pregnant.

For those committed to the prevention of problems and the promotion of competence, it is clearly necessary to address this level of advocacy directly. To accomplish this aspect of prevention programming, we learned that we must work with policymakers to raise their consciousness, increase understanding of the adverse impact of some policies, and demonstrate the potential of prevention services. To approach these goals at the social policy level requires an assertive presentation of our views, the views of prevention constituents, and the results of tested programs to those in power. We can also help formulate and implement policy. By integrating applied research techniques, we can design prevention programs that are testable and that provide evidence of their consequences. A successful policy argument integrates emotion, evidence, and action. The prevention planner should handle each of these aspects, and our model provides a frame-work for that effort.

CONCLUSION

The very first lesson that we learned from our experience was that prevention is much broader in scope and more complicated than the original program designs imagined. There are many levels of change involved, and many different elements to coordinate. Failure to understand this complexity and to plan for interactions will severely restrict prevention success. We have learned over 15 years that although an intervention may have a proven impact at one level, the program is unlikely to be sustained over time if the intervention is restricted to this one level. A proven individual change technique, for example, needs an effective organizational change plan to institutionalize its use. Furthermore, many interventions have natural implications for other levels that may prove unsuccessful if not carefully planned. A program for caregivers, for example, can create pressures for organizational change, whereas one for parents may require flexibility by teachers.

The most basic lesson that we have tried to convey conceptually and with a few examples is that prevention/promotion in mental health can be done. Such interventions can be successful with our current state of knowledge if programming involves stake-holders and constituents, and plans clearly to respond to the needs of the variety of levels essential to such programs.

References

Brager, G., & Holloway, S. (1978) *Changing human service organizations.* New York: Free Press.

Broskowski, A., & Baker, F. (1974). Professional, organizational, and social barriers to primary prevention. *American Journal of Orthopsychiatry, 45,* 707-719.

Caplan, G., & Grunebaum, H. (1967). Perspectives on primary prevention. *Archives of General Psychiatry.*

Chilman, C. S. (1966). *Growing up poor.* Washington, DC: USDHEW.

Cowen, E. L. (1982). *The special number: A complete road-map.* Paper presented at a Mini-Conference on Primary Prevention, Austin, Texas, Sponsored by NIMH, Office of Prevention.

Felner, R., Ginter, M, & Primivera, J. (1982). Primary prevention structure during school transitions: Social support and environmental structure. *American Journal of Community Psychology 10,* 277-290.

Forquer, S. (1981/1982). Planning primary prevention programs: A practical model. *Journal of Children in Contemporary Society, 14.*

Glasscote, R., Fishman, H., Sonis, M. (1972). *Services for children in mental health centers.* Washington, DC: American Psychiatric Association.

Goldston, S. (1977). *An overview of primary prevention programming.* Washington, DC: NIMH, Office of Prevention.

Hall, C. (1983). *A model for state-wide prevention planning in Connecticut.* Position paper, Office of Prevention.

Hermalin, J., & Weirich, T. W. (1982). Prevention research in field settings: A guide for practitioners. *Prevention in Human Services, 3.*

Hollister, W. G. (1976). *Basic strategies in designing primary prevention programs.* Pilot Conference on Primary Prevention, Philadelphia.

In Pursuit of Wellness, (1979). California Department of Mental Health, Office of Prevention.

Johnson, J., Healey, K., & Swift, M. (1981). Burnout prevention training for school administrators. *Stress, 2,* 15-19.

Klein, D. C., & Goldston, S. E. (Eds.). (1976). *Primary prevention: An idea whose time has come.* Washington, DC: NIMH.

Litwak, E. (1971). An approach to linkage in "grass roots" community organization. In F. Cox, J. Rothman, & J. Tropman (Eds.), *Strategies of community organization* (pp. 126-138). Itasca, IL: Peacock.

Lorion, R. (1984). A survey of prevention programs: Issues for consumers *Division of Community Psychology Newsletter.*

Nadler, D. A. (1981a). Managing organizational change: An Integrative perspective. *Journal of Applied Behavorial Science, 17,* 191-211.

Nadler, D. A. (1981b). *The planning and design approach.* New York: John Wiley.

National Institute of Mental Health. (1973). *Evaluation of the impact of community mental health centers.* Washington, DC: Author.

Spivack, G., & Swift, M. (1977). High-risk classroom behaviors in kindergarten and first grades. *American Journal of Community Psychology, 5.*

Swift, M. (1970). Training poverty mothers in communication skills. *The Reading Teacher, 23,* 360-367.

Swift, M. (1976a). *Some significant issues in training mental health clinicians in consultation and education.* Hahnemann Community Mental Health Center Report.

Swift, M. (1976b). *Education for prevention in a community mental health setting.* Hahnemann University Mental Health Center Report.

Tallman, I. (1976). *Passion, action, and politics.* San Francisco: W. H. Freeman.

Van de Ven, A. H. (1980). Problem solving, planning, and innovation. Part I. Test of the program planning model. *Human Relations 33,* 757-779.

Van de Ven, A. H., & Koenig, R. A. (1976). A process model for program planning and evaluation. *Journal of Economics and Business, 28,* 161-170.

Weirich, T. W., & Hermalin, J. A. (1982). Collaborative research in primary prevention: The practitioner-research relationship. In F. D. Perlmutter (Ed.), *New directions for mental health services.* San Francisco: Jossey-Bass.

Weirich, T. W., & Perlmutter, F. D. (1977, December). Interorganizational behavior patterns of line staff and services integration. *Social Service Review,* pp. 674-689.

Chapter 3

PREVENTION PLANNING AT THE FEDERAL LEVEL

STEPHEN E. GOLDSTON

Within the federal establishment, planning is a continuous ongoing process. Various requirements and dicta from higher levels mandate that material be prepared for comprehensive planning documents (for Institute, agency, Public Health Service, Department, and sometimes the Congress). The time frames involved frequently differ; whereas one requirement may be for a plan covering a five-year period, another plan may be limited to a fiscal year, six months, or even less. Plans are rarely reliable over time, that is, one year's plan may bear little similarity to material prepared a year hence or the previous year. In short, plans are not promises or commitments to be implemented lest some penalty be extracted.

In the event the reader senses some cynical view of planning reflected in the paragraph above, I hasten to indicate such was not my intent. Rather, I wish to state at the outset that (1) plans are not set in concrete to be executed as proposed or even sometimes followed through on at all, (2) fields of forces change

Author's Note: The views expressed in this chapter are mine and do not necessarily reflect the official position of the National Institute of Mental Health or any other part of the U.S. Department of Health and Human Services.

even over short periods of time, and these forces have an effect on planning, and (3) there often appears to be no end to requests for material to be supplied for this or that planning document. It took me a long time to learn what has been stated above. For quite some time I had believed that planning was purposive in that the energies devoted to planning were directly related to efforts to be expended to implement that plan. I am wiser now. At best, plans are guides.

This chapter contains a brief history of planning efforts at the National Institute of Mental Health to develop a formal federal prevention program. Having served as the only professional staff member assigned full-time to prevention program development, or, to put it in federal-ese, having been the lead person for prevention from 1967 to 1979, and then from 1981 to the present, the telling of this history is inextricably interwoven with personal views, values, and reflections. This comment is set forth both as a caveat for the reader to remain alert to possible idiosyncratic interpretations, and to affirm that it is rarely possible for one to be a part of history making without having influenced the direction and nature of that history and also having strong passions about the issues involved.

EARLY FEDERAL PREVENTION PLANNING

The year 1974 is a good starting point for examining the federal role in preventive mental health planning. That year two documents of major significance were released, one by the federal government in Canada and the other by the U.S. government. The Canadian document, titled *A New Perspective on the Health of Canadians,* issued in the name of Marc Lalonde (1975), then Minister of National Health and Welfare, and subsequently to be referred to as the "Lalonde Report," expounded the following fundamental position: "Future improvements in the level of health of Canadians lie mainly in improving the environment, moderating self-imposed risks and adding to our knowledge of human biology" (p. 18). The report went on: "There is the paradox of everyone agreeing to the importance of research and prevention yet continuing to increase disproportionally the amount of money spent on treating existing illness [p. 30]. . . . It is apparent therefore, that vast sums are being spent treating diseases that could have been prevented in the first place" (p. 32).

Two months after release of the Lalonde Report, in June 1974, the U.S. Department of Health, Education, and Welfare (DHEW) issued its first *Forward Plan for Health* for the five-year period FY 1976-1980. Among the five themes in the plan, prevention was listed first, a ranking of no small significance given that prevention in the past had rarely been discussed in any federal health document. This plan, inclusive of both physical health and mental health, stated that "preventing illness, injury and premature death must be a major component of this Nation's health strategy. . . a fundamental component of our emphasis on prevention is a full commitment to research, evaluation, and the generation of new knowledge. . . prevention not only alleviates human suffering, it also holds the key to the lock on our present and foreseeable health care problems, including their costs" (p. 7). The similarity in tone and direction of these two documents is no less remarkable than the boldness of their statements on behalf of the unequivocable, explicit support of prevention.

In addition to the general statements on prevention, the DHEW plan also contained specific content about prevention in mental health.

(1) One goal in our mental health strategy for FY 1976-80 is to extend services beyond the traditional direct methods of treating persons in need and to mobilize the concern of the community in providing effective programs of prevention of mental illness.
(2) Our preventive thrusts will include not only the diagnosed illnesses such as schizophrenia and depression or the more recently, more clearly defined areas of alcoholism and drug abuse, but will extend as far as possible to addressing such social stresses as the influence of violence on television, racism, crime and delinquency, poverty, and suicide.
(3) Special initiatives will place specific emphasis on family

problems. These efforts will be directed at such problems as child abuse and neglect, and youth who run away from home. Minority group mental health problems and metropolitan mental health problems are two more areas which will be dealt with in a preventive perspective.

(4) In coping with the preventive aspect of mental health in all of these high-risk groups, continuing research for identifying needs, providing a sound basis of information, and formulating agency policy will be stressed. (pp. 32-33)

Finally, the 1974 document specified the following NIMH prevention plans:

NIMH will continue its prevention activities through direct community mental health services, such as emergency and crisis management, outpatient outreach services, and medical and psychotherapeutic aftercare. Research and evaluation of consultation and education and community care programs will be supported to distinguish which interactions have most impact on the populations.

In addition NIMH will give priority to programs concerned with prevention of impairment in children and youth through early detection, management of developmental and situational crises, through training in coping skills, and through the study of effective developmental environments. Attention will also be given to increasing personal effectiveness and development of coping skills among teachers. The NIMH preventive thrusts will also include the diagnosed illnesses, such as schizophrenia and depression, and areas such as racism, crime and delinquency, poverty, and suicide. (p. 89)

Two matters merit note. First, it was planners in the *physical* health sphere that included mental health in their report. Second, the form of prevention being addressed clearly was not *primary* prevention, but explicitly secondary prevention (early diagnosis and treatment) and tertiary prevention (rehabilitation). Nonetheless, the important fact is that in June 1974 prevention appeared officially on the DHEW agenda as a priority theme for health planning and implementation. In brief, the 1974 plan provided prevention with an official sanction for the first time.

Although I have chosen 1974 as the year when mental health prevention planning efforts began, actually by that time NIMH already had a history of planning efforts concerned with advancing prevention and mental health promotion. In early 1968, several months after being named as Special Assistant to the Director for Preventive Programs, I prepared at the request of the director of NIMH a staff working paper that called for a National Center for the Prevention of Mental Illness and the Promotion of Mental Health (Goldston, 1968). The official response to that document was to invite a panel of experts to provide advice to NIMH about primary prevention. Thus, in June 1968, a prestigious group of mental health workers (including George Albee, Eli Bower, Leonard Duhl, Reginald Lourie, John Clausen, and Julius Richmond) constituted a consultant panel to advise NIMH on program development in primary prevention, including program strategies and specific proposals.

The Prevention Panel met three times and in March 1970 sent to the director of NIMH a report entitled *Promoting Mental Health*. Having reviewed the extent of NIMH's efforts in primary prevention the Panel concluded, "NIMH's current involvement in primary prevention activities is *underdeveloped and unfocused*" [emphasis added]. The Panel advocated a primary prevention program for NIMH including specific priority areas (namely, activities related to early child development and to increased parental competence, and programs focused on the mental health aspects of public school education and adolescence), numerous programmatic functions, linkages with other key agencies and organizations, and an Institute self-study of ongoing primary prevention efforts. The Panel's report went on to state,

> Major gaps in program efforts in this area can be filled only by creating a specific program focus with sufficient budgetary

allocations... it would not seem unreasonable to consider building up to a level of support equal to approximately one-half of the NIMH budget.... The Panel proposes that an organizational structure and focal point be established within NIMH which would have visible responsibility and authority for programming in the area of primary prevention.

The report further indicated, "Assigned staff, adequate budget, clear lines of authority and responsibility, a defined relationship to other parts of NIMH, and a clear program mandate are required if NIMH determines to develop this area." The Panel concluded,

It is now timely and appropriate for NIMH to devote the same maximum effort of talent, energy, and resources which went into the community mental health centers program, schizophrenia research, manpower development, and hospital improvement toward a national program in primary prevention.

In spite of the compelling arguments put forth by the Panel, apparently in March 1970 primary prevention was not yet an idea whose time had come. The ideas advanced, in spite of the high-standing of their advocates and authors, were not sufficiently persuasive in terms of the political realities of that time to bring prevention to center stage, even given the relative modesty of most of the recommendations when translated into administrative structure, staffing, budget, and program. Somewhat similar recommendations put forth in 1975, 1976, and 1977 to establish a small administrative unit for primary prevention likewise were shelved and not acted upon favorably.

But I have digressed from the chronology of the story...

As indicated, the *Forward Plan for Health, FY 1976-80* (DHEW, 1974) provided initial official sanction for prevention. However, the following year's document, the *Forward Plan for Health, FY 1977-81,* issued in June 1975, was even more affirmative about prevention.

Once again, the plan included prevention as one of its major emphases or themes. The following statements attest to the importance invested in prevention by the planners:

(1) A basic premise of the prevention strategy (is) that much greater attention and resources must be directed at preventing the underlying causes of disease rather than at the disease itself.... Enough is known about the underlying causes to justify major preventive action now.... An overwhelming proportion of them (diseases) are caused by man and his institutions and can be controlled by man. (p. 16)

(2) Over the next several years, all programs of the Public Health Service will seek ways to concentrate their energies and talent on attacking the underlying causes of disease and on helping people and communities to take direct responsibility for protecting their own health. (p. 19)

(3) For planning purposes, we believe it is more productive to focus our attention on the underlying conditions or antecedent causes of preventable diseases than to concentrate on the diseases themselves. (p. 98)

With this comment, the U.S. report acknowledged indebtedness to the Lalonde Report.

(4) While we propose that a higher priority be given to the development of primary prevention programs directed at the underlying causes of disease, we recognize that in some instances our capacity to affect these problems is limited or unknown. Many of them involve fundamental changes in the behavior of people and in the traditional practices of social and economic institutions. It would be unrealistic to expect significant improvements within a short time. Efforts will therefore continue to be directed toward improving the scope and utility of prevention programs for the early detection and treatment of disease and for the reduction of disability and dependence. This must be accompanied by an assessment of the efficacy and costs of all preventive approaches. (p. 98)

Finally, a mention of primary prevention, but followed quickly by a "safe retreat" back to secondary and tertiary prevention approaches. But wait, the report continues:

(5) A basic assumption underlying our approach is that despite major gaps in our knowledge, enough is known about the

links between these diseases and their antecedent conditions
to justify a special emphasis on *primary prevention action
now.* (emphasis added; p. 99)

That statement afforded an endorsement for primary prevention; the next paragraph was virtually a "Magna Carta" for
prevention:

(6) Perhaps more important at this time than agreement on
specific proposals is the explicit *commitment* of the Public
Health Service and the Secretary of HEW to the goals of
primary prevention and the determination to apply the energies and resources of this Department to help find practical
ways of achieving those goals. (emphasis added; p. 99)

To those of us who viewed ourselves as "true believers" in
primary prevention, this statement was met with a sense of
enthusiasm and redemption. There was also hope that the long-
awaited opportunity to secure resources and to pursue the
legitimate activities characterizing "established" programs (i.e.,
research, training, and service projects) finally would be accorded
to primary prevention. However, as events demonstrated, in a
large bureaucracy even word from the highest echelons requires
time both to reach the operating units below and to be acted
upon after the message has been received.

The 1975 report went on to state some specific options for
mental health action, including developing mental health programs focused on helping individuals to cope with life crises,
increasing communications between mental health programs and
a variety of human services agencies, and supporting research
on preventing developmental failures in children.

Lastly, the following material about NIMH prevention activities appeared in the report:

Since its inception, NIMH has emphasized the importance of
understanding the basis of, and promoting, positive mental health
as well as the importance of being concerned with the etiology,
incidence, and treatment of mental illness. However, activities

related to prevention have for the most part been developed and carried out within a variety of programs ranging from basic studies on the relation of culture to identity formation, or early infant stimulating and cognitive development, to demonstration projects to improve the "climate" of early child care centers and schools.

Thus, while the Institute's involvement in prevention has been extensive, it has also been *undirected and unfocused.* A major Institute objective for the planning period is to bring organized thinking and program planning to bear on its prevention-related efforts. (emphasis added; pp. 250-251)

From a historical perspective, we should note that almost a decade after the Prevention Panel's report (1970) and five years following the initial departmental planning report (1974), the first administrative structure for prevention, the Office of Prevention, was established at NIMH in fall 1979. In April 1982, three years later, as part of an overall Institute reorganization, the research grant responsibilities and authority of the Office of Prevention were transferred to a newly created, second administrative unit for prevention, the Prevention Research Branch, which several months later was renamed the Center for Prevention Research.

The creation of the first administrative structure for prevention program development was a major achievement. In bureaucracies, official designation of form and function invariably precedes the allocation of fiscal and staff resources. With the establishment of the Office of Prevention, the area of prevention achieved legitimacy and the opportunity to pursue programmatic goals and objectives.

Given the lengthy history eventuating in bureaucratic sanction for prevention, one might inquire about what happened to all the products generated during the planning exercises and efforts conducted from 1968 onward. My experience as a planner attests analogously to the physical law that matter can neither be created nor destroyed, that is, good prevention ideas have a timelessness. The burdens of the human condition, be they the harmful consequences of marital disruption, bereavement, having a psychotic parent, raising a malformed child, or whatever, continue. Accordingly, I filed the reports and ideas not in a wastebasket but in accessible places, knowing that the time would come when these plans could be promoted once again, at a time when the political tides and the field of forces would have been sufficiently modified so as to favor prevention approaches and programs.

From the experience of prevention advocacy and the preparation of planning documents for over two decades, some lessons for planners emerge:

(1) Good ideas are not necessarily new ideas; some proposals continue to have merit long after their origination.
(2) Many good ideas have yet to be translated into acceptable practices in communities across the nation. For example, in spite of all the research demonstrating the positive results of psychological preparation of children and their families in connection with hospitalization for a medical or surgical condition, most hospitals serving pediatric patients do not have formal preparation programs.
(3) The truth of Ecclesiastes remains pertinent—"for everything there is a season." Ideas cannot be born and implemented before their time. A critical mass of support, scientific background, and temper of the times must be in harmony.
(4) Perseverance is essential.

The preceding background information brings us to the starting point of where NIMH was from a program perspective when prevention became an official, mandated activity within the Public Health Service and the then Department of Health, Education, and Welfare. We move to an in-depth look at how prevention plans were developed at NIMH and how they were implemented or otherwise.

THE DEVELOPMENT OF MENTAL HEALTH PREVENTION INITIATIVES

In December 1977 an intensive planning effort focused on prevention began within the Public Health Service under the leadership of the Office of the Assistant Secretary for Health/ Surgeon General. Composed of staff from the various PHS components, three work groups gathered information about each agency's prevention efforts, identified gaps, and recommended new prevention programs as related to the elements of lifestyle, environment, and personal preventive health services. The products of these work groups provided the comprehensive information compiled in the report *Healthy People* issued in 1979.

During the same time frame, a planning process was initiated within the Alcohol, Drug Abuse, and Mental Health Administration that was based on the following conceptualization of prevention:

(1) Mental Health Promotion—improving coping capacity and competence, for example, facilitating sound parent-infant mental health.

(2) Disease/Disorder Prevention—specific protection against disease and disorders, for example, acute and chronic brain syndromes.

(3) Prevention of Behavioral Consequences—interventions to prevent the deleterious effects (consequences) of high-risk behaviors, for example, accidents resulting from drinking while driving, suicide as a consequence of emotional disorders or excessive drinking or substance abuse.

(4) Prevention of Behavioral Antecedents—interventions to prevent high-risk behaviors that are conditions precedent to physical, emotional, and behavioral problems, for example, heavy teenage drinking, smoking, experimental drug use.

Importantly, this framework defined prevention as primary prevention; the focus was to be on specific population groups that had not been diagnosed as psychiatrically disturbed.

The proposed outcome of this planning process was for each of the component agencies of the Alcohol, Drug Abuse, and Mental Health Administration (ADAMHA), that is, the National Institute of Mental Health (NIMH), the National Institute for Drug Abuse (NIDA), and the National Institute for Alcohol Abuse and Alcoholism (NIAAA), to specify new prevention programs (or initiatives). The guidelines for planning called for the initiatives to be formulated in terms of specific goals, measurable objectives (both long- and short-term), evaluation procedures, and resources required for program development. Further, proposed initiatives were to be data-based.

Within NIMH, prevention planning—from the identification of initiatives through their future implementation—was devised in terms of overall program development. By definition, a program was seen as a "cluster of related, specific, commonly shared goal-oriented activities, in distinction to disparate projects" (Goldston, 1979). Thus an attempt was made to build into the planning the objective of arriving at initiatives aimed at specific targeted problem solving of major mental health/public health concerns as distinguished from merely advocating projects that focused on a single part or aspect of the total problem but having little effect on the overall problem area. In other words, only multifaceted initiatives were acceptable.

Additionally, each proposed initiative was to focus on a specific problem area meeting the needs of a specific population for specific stated purposes. Multiple strategy elements were to be included with each initiative, for example, research, services demonstration, health education and information, capacity-building at the state and community levels, and opportunities for technology transfer, that is, providing information on a continuous basis during the time of the initiative.

Program development was guided by two other conditions: (a) fiscal realities, and (b) the need to identify initiatives that could achieve within a stated time period the measurable goals, thus demonstrating the relevance and effectiveness of primary prevention approaches.

A major guiding principle in initiative development was to identify opportunities for intervention in order to meet the objectives of either (a) reducing the incidence of dysfunction or disorder, or (b) promoting optimal psychological functioning. Accordingly, the proposed initiatives were to be formulated as opportunities for the development and evaluation of intervention models. An initial goal would be to ascertain what works, to develop the models; "The ultimate goal would be the delivery of services to people in need, after field trials had indicated the efficacy of the models" (Goldston, 1979).

In early February 1978, a prevention planning process began within NIMH for the purpose of identifying initiatives within the guidelines cited above. Each of the operating divisions was requested through their director to complete a form providing information about proposed initiatives. I met individually with each division director to clarify the nature of the task and his or her responsibility for preparing proposals for new and/or expanded initiatives. By the receipt deadline two weeks later, 51 initiative statements had been submitted. From this total, 9 were omitted due to excessive vagueness in the writeup or non-applicability to the stated task. The remaining 42 initiatives were reviewed, edited to conform to a prescribed format, and compiled into a "compendium" of initiatives. Within this compendium the initiatives were grouped into 5 thematic areas: children and youth, families, crises of death/bereavement/loss, epidemiology of vulnerable populations, and mobilization of existing community support systems as a preventive mental health resource.

This compendium was then forwarded to each division director and to members of the Institute acting director's immediate staff requesting comments. The next step was to compile a draft document that identified those initiatives most appropriate to the guidelines for the stated task, namely, initiatives that dealt with research, the development of demonstration intervention models within a research framework, and information gathering and dissemination. The 16 initiatives that made the cut were reviewed by the Institute acting director in consultation with staff; the list was pared down to 6 initiatives based on conformance to the ADAMHA planning guidelines, the strength of the existing data bases, and the likelihood of demonstrating program effectiveness within a three- to five-year support period. The 6 initiatives in the plan to begin in Fiscal Year 1980 included the following:

- To foster the mental health of children experiencing the stressful life event of hospitalization

- To enhance the mental health of parents and infants by means of coordinated mental health promotion interventions
- To promote effective coping among family members experiencing the stress of marital separation/divorce
- To promote the capacity of the American people to cope with the crisis of death in the family
- To develop and extend effective mental health prevention programs to communities stricken by major disasters
- To ascertain variables contributing to the marked increase in suicidal behavior among high-risk persons (ages 10-24 years and 65 and over) and develop prevention-intervention programs to ameliorate this condition.

In addition to the 6 initiatives scheduled to be implemented in October 1979, four other initiatives were included to be phased in during subsequent years on such topics as children of severely disturbed/institutionalized parents, state-level primary prevention offices, psychosocial aspects of chronic illness, and establishing an NIMH R&D Primary Prevention Center.

At this point, some comments on the dynamics operating during the planning process appear appropriate because they tend to be of general applicability. Within bureaucracies, new sources of funds often are perceived as "fair game" for existing, established programs. In this instance, the operating divisions, having been requested to submit prevention proposals, were reminded that prevention was part of their program mission; as a result, the prevention proposals forthcoming from such administrative subunits tended to be characterized more by the culture and values of that group than by the stipulated guidelines. For example, whereas the prevention planning process mandated that the focus was to be on primary prevention, a significant number of the proposals submitted dealt with secondary and tertiary prevention, for example, secondary and tertiary prevention of severe functional mental disorders, prevention of adverse consequences of psychotherapeutic drug use, and prevention of relapse in schizophrenic and affective disordered patients in the community. A few proposals related to basic research that at best might be classified as prevention-related or of prevention-potential, for example, studies of the fundamental biological processes of the major mental disorders, and epidemiological studies of the risk factors associated with the incidence of specific mental disorders. In addition, there was little tradition to fall back on with respect to prevention—no official definitions, no clear consensus as to what grants in the overall research portfolio might be labeled prevention, and little staff expertise in prevention. Such conditions tend to contribute toward conflict and open competition for new funds; at minimum, staff tensions can arise requiring considerable goodwill and interprofessional respect in order to facilitate the birthing process for a new program.

In mid-March 1978, ADAMHA staff issued a memorandum spelling out the framework for preparation of a formal document containing the prevention plan. This specific framework contained the following elements: background and history of each Institute's prevention program, proposed program for the period Fiscal Year 1977-1982, and the new and continuing initiatives planned for implementation in Fiscal Year 1980-1982. The latter item referred to the new prevention plan and requested information on the following matters: description of the initiatives and the relationship to overall Institute goals, the objectives to be accomplished, research and other data that provide the knowledge base for the initiatives, time frame for phasing the initiatives over a 3-year period, the strategies to be utilized, the evaluation plan, and costs. Less than 10 working days were provided to submit the plan.

By the close of March, the NIMH plan was submitted to the Institute acting director for final review prior to being forwarded to the administrator of ADAMHA. In the covering memo prepared in sending the plan to the Institute acting director, I made some comments relevant to planners as well as historians of prevention. The memo pointed out some reasons why the plan fell short of adequately meeting the challenge of prevention:

(1) The development of the plan was shaped by the imperatives of the guidelines and the need to identify new initiatives. This approach precluded the development of a plan in which the

initiatives were a part rather than the totality. In sum, the planning process called for goals, objectives, and, it was hoped, administrative structures to emerge from the initiatives, whereas a more productive approach would have had the initiatives emanate from prior considerations about goals, objectives, and structures.

(2) New structures, new mechanisms, and new approaches were required to develop and implement the prevention plan. Of the six initiatives, four were demonstration programs with training, research, and service elements interwoven therein. No single existing NIMH administrative component was an appropriate location for such program development in view of the limits of their stated missions. Moreover, to decentralize responsibility for these initiatives or portions thereof among more than one existing component would not serve to advance the fledgling prevention effort.

(3) The plan contained no mechanisms for coordinating current and/or ongoing prevention activities.

(4) The plan did not represent an overall NIMH approach to the many opportunities for prevention. Many key problems and groups at risk were not included in the plan. Further, the involvements in prevention by existing NIMH units remained unclear.

(5) The prevention plan called for funds to become available in October 1980, but no funds or mechanisms were indicated for preparatory work during an 18-month interim period.

(6) The plan provided no opportunities for further prevention program development beyond the six initiatives during the period Fiscal Year 1980-1982.

Critique aside, this memo stated that the plan represented a new approach to program development, an active, problem-oriented approach attempting to deal with some major mental health/public health matters in an integrated fashion. Further, some of the initiatives proposed to have an impact on national issues and attitudes whereas other initiatives would test out hypotheses and acquire new knowledge as a forerunner of extending intervention efforts across the nation. In closing, I noted prophetically, "We are still only at the beginning."

During the months immediately following submission of the NIMH prevention plan in March 1978, planning activities continued. The originally identified prevention initiatives were subsequently reworked and revised to be consistent with the following factors:

(1) The recommendations forthcoming from the President's Commission on Mental Health.
(2) The need to have the emerging prevention plan reflect both the range of prevailing views about prevention as well as the capacity of the field to act.
(3) The inclusion in the President's FY 80 budget of a $6 million item for research on prevention.
(4) The importance of developing an NIMH-wide prevention program that involved all the major Institute components.

By the close of calendar year 1978, the NIMH prevention plan had three programmatic elements:

(1) Research Initiatives. Seven research initiatives were developed, each addressed to a specific major health/public health problem. Every initiative was to include various research strategies in order to develop demonstration intervention models; the ultimate objective was obtaining information needed for the more effective delivery services to persons in need. The specific initiatives include the mental health of children experiencing the stressful life event of hospitalization, parental competency, the stress of marital separation/divorce, pathological grief reactions, community disasters, suicidal behavior, and the effects of severe parental mental disorder on vulnerable children.

(2) Service Initiatives. Anticipating passage of the Mental Health Systems Act and the allocation of funds for prevention service projects, four service initiatives were identified, including the development of intervention models for identified underserved, high-risk groups, an experimental epidemiology project, support for the establishment of state-level offices of primary prevention, and a prevention information storage/retrieval system.

(3) R&D Primary Prevention Capacity. The proposed R&D capacity involved the creation of an administrative locus within NIMH for (a) managing the research and service initiatives, (b) coordinating other NIMH prevention efforts, (c) supporting new promising prevention research and demonstration projects, (d) developing a primary prevention training academy, (e) conducting primary prevention program development workshops, and (f) developing extramural field stations and centers of excellence for prevention research.

Let us review the outcomes of planning, looking back on an almost seven-year period, extending from March 1978 to the beginning of calendar year 1985 when this chapter was in preparation.

THE OUTCOMES OF PREVENTION PLANNING

In order to implement any plan, certain basic elements must be present—administrative structures and mechanisms, and allocated resources, including dollars and staff. Therefore, as a preface to our discussion of the outcomes of prevention planning, it is critical to note that by the fall of 1979, NIMH had made a firm programmatic and policy commitment to prevention. That commitment was translated into action by the establishment of the Office of Prevention within the Office of the Director of NIMH and the allocation of $4 million as a specific budget item for prevention. The mission statement for the Office of Prevention identified the following functions:

- serving as the NIMH lead for activities related to the prevention of mental illness and the promotion of mental health;
- coordinating and developing Institutewide policies for prevention goals, priorities, and programs;
- stimulating, developing, supporting, and monitoring activities including developing and convening planning workshops, commissioning key technical and advisory reports, preparing and disseminating relevant prevention information, initiating and facilitating policy studies, and arranging expert consultations;
- initiating and fostering liaison and collaborative efforts with

federal, state, regional, and local agencies, voluntary organizations, public and private educational agencies, and organizations representing service providers, scientific groups, and service consumers to facilitate program development;
- identifying, analyzing, and evaluating current research and related program developments in the area of prevention, directing this information to citizens, administrators, and policymakers as an aid for assessing policy and action alternatives;
- identifying specific areas of opportunity for strategic prevention planning and program development.

Further, Section 325 of the Mental Health Systems Act provided a legal mandate and sanction for prevention:

The Director [of NIMH] shall designate an administrative unit in the Institute to—(1) design national goals and establish national priorities for—(A) the prevention of mental illness, and (B) the promotion of mental health, (2) encourage and assist local entities and State agencies to achieve the goals and priorities described in paragraph (1), and (3) develop and coordinate Federal prevention policies and programs to assure increased focus on the prevention of mental illness and the promotion of mental health.

In August 1981, the Congress enacted the Omnibus Budget Reconciliation Act of 1981, which repealed the Mental Health Systems Act and authorized block grants to the states. Among the four sections of that act that were not repealed was Section 325, entitled "National Institute of Mental Health Prevention Unit," now designated Section 455(d) of the Public Health Service Act. The Office of Prevention is responsible for the planning effort and related program implementation required to carry out the provisions of this legislation.

By fall 1981 a total NIMH reorganization process had begun. As indicated earlier in this chapter, one result was the creation of a prevention research unit charged with research program development and administration of prevention intervention research grants, formerly the responsibility of the Office of Prevention. In April 1982, this new administrative unit, the Center for Prevention Research, was established within the newly named Division of Prevention and Special Mental Health Programs.

In fiscal year 1983, $8.7 million was expanded for prevention research grants (Alcohol, Drug Abuse, and Mental Health Administration [ADAMHA], 1984, p. 19). With respect to staffing, the Center for Prevention Research had the approximate equivalent of six full-time professionals, and the Office of Prevention, one full-time professional.

To a large extent, the two administrative units for prevention within NIMH have functioned to address satisfactorily the proposed initiative calling for an R&D Primary Prevention Capacity. The Center for Prevention Research (a) manages research initiatives; with NIMH's former service activities block granted to the states, there are no service initiatives, (b) supports new promising prevention research; no authorization exists for demonstration projects, and (c) develops centers of excellence for prevention research, namely, the Prevention Intervention Research Centers (PIRCs) being supported by NIMH. By the close of fiscal year 1984, five such centers had been funded; no extramural field stations were planned or developed. The Office of Prevention (a) coordinates nonresearch NIMH prevention efforts, and (b) conducts prevention program development workshops. The proposal to establish a primary prevention training academy was not acted on, largely due to the overall annual uncertainties with respect to funding for clinical training. On balance, the proposed functions to be provided by an R&D primary prevention capacity within NIMH have been addressed through the two established prevention units.

The major prevention planning activity pursued by the Office of Prevention has involved a series of workshops initiated during fiscal year 1981. From the outset, the research planning workshops were perceived as an integral step in program development. Operationally, these workshops were 2.5-day invitational meetings in which 12 to 14 experts came together around a specific content issue. The tasks for the experts included the following: identifying both the state-of-the-art of research knowledge on that specific content area and the gaps in knowledge, determining the readiness of the field for preventive interventions, prioritizing a research agenda, and preparing recommendations to NIMH. In those areas where it was determined that the field was ready for research on preventive interventions, when conditions warranted, the notion was that funds would be set aside and program announcements be forthcoming inviting applications in that specific content area. In addition, proceedings documents and other publications were to be products of the workshops.

The workshop mechanism has been used to accomplish several purposes: (1) to identify major parts of the "cutting edge" of prevention research, (2) to develop a means of proceeding from expert planning and input to the actual support of innovative research, (3) to involve and enlist a constituency of senior researchers who would both be encouraged to undertake prevention research and be supportive of such efforts, and (4) to produce documents in connection with the NIMH Prevention Publication Series.

With the transfer of prevention research functions to the Center for Prevention Research, the Office of Prevention convened state-of-the-art workshops and technical assistance workshops aimed at addressing specific prevention issues relating to services, information transfer, and other nonresearch program development concerns.

The workshops convened from fiscal year 1981 through fiscal year 1984 looked at many aspects of prevention, including the media, American Indian and Alaska Native communities, stress-related psychiatric disorders, severe and persistent loneliness, psychiatric epidemiology, families with a mentally ill relative, cost-effectiveness and cost-offset research, suicide and affective disorders among adolescents, childhood chronic illness, disabling anger, depression, ethics, healthy family functioning, aggressive and violent behavior, and black homicide. Participants have indicated that their involvement in the workshops resulted in a significant increase in the extent to which their activities include prevention.

We turn now to review the outcomes of the research initiatives proposed in 1978. In actuality, only research funds became available; therefore, the notion of developing demonstration intervention models that included the elements of research, training, and services was set aside. Of the original seven initiatives proposed, only two have contributed directly toward the planned purpose of program model development—the initiatives on (1) promoting effective coping among family members experiencing the stress of marital separation/divorce, and (2) minimizing the deleterious effects of severe parental mental disorder on vulnerable children. For each of these initiatives, special announcements were prepared and distributed to the field in fiscal year 1980, inviting applications dealing with preventive intervention research and new knowledge development on (a) the impact of marital disruption on children, and (b) the effects on children of having a severely disturbed parent, whether mentally or emotionally ill, alcoholic, or drug abuser. At this writing, a consolidated report is being prepared on the research supported in connection with the marital disruption initiative, while final data analyses are being conducted on the studies supported under the second initiative.

Activities pursued in connection with the other five proposed initiatives may be summarized as follows: (1) a contract was negotiated to develop an instrument to be used for a survey of mental health practices in pediatric settings; the instrument was produced, but the proposed survey to obtain national baseline data has not been conducted; (2) the specific initiative on parental competency that also related to preventing postpartum disturbances was not performed; (3) the initiative on death and bereavement resulted not in intervention research but in a research literature review study of the health consequences of the stress of bereavement (Osterweis, Solomon, & Green, 1984). I hope that this review will serve as the stimulus for a special announcement inviting applications on preventive interventions to deal with the harmful consequences of bereavement; (4) during the 1981-1982 NIMH reorganization, an administrative unit on emergency mental health was established; to date, no preventive intervention studies have been conducted; and (5) a suicide research unit was created within NIMH in 1983; to date, studies have focused on basic research, not preventive interventions.

As for the service initiatives, with repeal of the Mental Health Systems Act, funds were not forthcoming to support the proposed activities. However, considerable effort has been devoted to one of the four original service initiatives, namely, working with the various states to encourage prevention efforts. Related activities include the following: convening meetings of state prevention office directors, holding workshops on prevention for state commissioners of mental health, providing technical assistance to states on prevention matters, distributing prevention documents, and conducting a regional conference of prevention contracts from the 16 western states. Another service initiative that remains unfulfilled is the need to develop a formal information storage/retrieval system on prevention.

In summary, much of the original prevention planning package was carried through to implementation, though not always in the form proposed.

CONCLUDING REMARKS

It is time for some personal reflections and observations. I believe that good, meaningful planning should reflect operationally the vision one holds on how events should unfold in the development of a program area. For the advocates of prevention, that vision has been an imperative. Perhaps these guidelines may be useful to other planners:

(1) Things rarely turn out as planned. Had the prevention plan unfolded as proposed, the field of prevention would be significantly more advanced and more understood than is now the case. For instance, program manuals and other how-to documents would be available for service deliverers setting forth a variety of research-tested, data-based approaches to the development of prevention services. The need remains, and must be addressed.

(2) You can't control all the variables. The field of forces is in constant motion; the key players change. You can only plan based on the knowns and a liberal sprinking of the elements of your vision.

(3) Just because you believe, and the top person says "go," doesn't ensure smooth planning or program implementation in the manner proposed. Agendas conflict in the presence of finite budgets.

(4) Perseverance, tenacity, a good support system, a politically active constituency, and some research evidence can help a planner go a long way toward making a vision a reality.

References

Alcohol, Drug Abuse, and Mental Health Administration. (1984). *Prevention activities of the Alcohol, Drug Abuse, and Mental Health Administration—fiscal year 1983 report to Congress.* Rockville, MD: Author.

Goldston, S. E. (1968). *Proposal for a national center for the prevention of mental illness and the promotion of mental health.* Unpublished manuscript.

Goldston, S. E. (1979). Primary prevention programming from the federal perspective: A progress report. *Journal of Clinical Child Psychology, 8,* 80-83.

Lalonde, M. (1975). *A new perspective on the health of Canadians: A working document, April 1974.* Ottawa, Canada: Information Canada.

National Institute of Mental Health. (1970). *Promoting mental health.* Unpublished manuscript.

Osterweis, M., Solomon, F., & Green, M. (Eds.). (1984). *Bereavement: Reactions, consequences, and care.* Washington, DC: National Academy Press.

U.S. Department of Health, Education, and Welfare. (1974). *Forward plan for health FY 1976-80.* Washington, DC: Government Printing Office.

U.S. Department of Health, Education, and Welfare. (1975). *Forward plan for health FY 1977-81* (DHEW Publication No. (OS) 76-50024). Washington, DC: Government Printing Office.

U.S. Department of Health, Education, and Welfare. (1979). *Healthy people: The Surgeon General's report on health promotion and disease prevention* (DHEW Publication No. (PHS) 79-55071). Washington, DC: Government Printing Office.

Chapter 4

PREVENTION PLANNING IN COMMUNITY MENTAL HEALTH CENTERS

CAROLYN SWIFT

This chapter considers preventive planning in community mental health centers (CMHCs) from a systems perspective. Planning preventive interventions from a CMHC base involves examining the needs and resources of the community and negotiating the concerns of multiple constituencies. There are three broad groups examined here for their roles in the prevention planning process: the CMHC itself, the local community, and various levels of government. The support of the governmental infrastructure— city, county, state, and federal legislative and regulatory bodies—is critical because these groups control access to target populations and funds.

The chapter begins with an overview of the planning process. This discussion includes a projection of prevention goals and methods as these relate to the realities of the community mental health environment over the next decade. Four basic issues that have an impact on planning are considered in a systems context: the priority of the prevention mission, the role of the CMHC prevention planner, sources of funding for CMHC prevention programs, and constituency building. The body of the chapter is devoted to an examination of the planning process.

The planning process is a key element in delivering effective preventive services from a CMHC base. Although prevention planning requires the formulation of prevention goals and the projection of methods and strategies to meet the goals, it is the process by which these goals and strategies are decided and programs implemented that determines the ultimate success of CMHC prevention programming. Because the CMHC is part of a larger system of health and human service delivery, and because its fortunes are inextricably linked to the economic, social, and political conditions that affect the nation, the goals and strategies selected by CMHC prevention planners in the next decade are likely to diverge in major ways from those prevalent in the 1960s and 1970s. These divergences are outlined below. Although national economic and political realities reduce the degrees of freedom of CMHC preventionists to choose among prevention goals, there is still wide latitude in targeting populations and designing programs relevant to local communities. It is in this process of meeting community needs within the larger context of national policies and priorities that the CMHC prevention planner can function most effectively.

Preventive activities have undergone a dramatic shift in the 1980s. This shift is seen across all aspects of the preventive enterprise: in the goals and methods selected, in the resources available, and the outcomes projected (Armstrong, 1985; Backer, Shifrin-Levine, & Erchul, 1983; Snow & Swift, 1985). CMHC prevention efforts in the 1960s and 1970s took the global goal of preventing mental illness and targeted entire communities for prevention efforts. The reality of CMHC operations today is that the economic resources, the political will, and the scientific knowledge base available are insufficient to prevent mental illness on a communitywide basis (Rich & Goldsmith, 1983). To gain the support of local economic and political leaders for prevention activities, CMHC planners are advised to project outcomes that are observable, predictable, and significant in the context of narrower, more specific target group concerns. The appropriate goal of prevention activities in CMHCs in the next decade is to reduce the incidence of specific disorders, in at-risk populations that have relevance to the CMHC clinical caseloads, using methods demonstrated to be effective.

The current CMHC arena is one of reduced funding, with increased demands for services for the chronically mentally ill. In this milieu, where prevention must compete with treatment for scarce resources, the prevention activities most likely to receive support fall into three categories. First, prevention activities that are consonant with, or augment, services that benefit CMHC clinical clients or their families are more likely to receive support from CMHC administrators, citizen boards, and patient advocacy groups (Rich & Goldsmith, 1983; Tableman, 1984). Children of the chronically mentally ill, or those with alcoholic, drug-dependent, or divorced parents are major at-risk populations. Interventions with these groups satisfy both solid prevention aims and the clinical needs associated with their parents' treatment.

A second set of prevention activities focuses on specific disorders that result in moderate to severe disruptions in large numbers of community residents (Rich & Goldsmith, 1983). Examples here include a variety of stress-related illnesses with both physical and behavioral components—such as heart disease—and illnesses of special concern to specific communities—such as those resulting from exposure to toxic chemicals from local industries. The third set of prevention activities likely to win support over the next decade involves disorders that constitute a crisis within the ecology of the community as well as the host population. Teenage pregnancy is an example of a social problem that has a major impact on community resources and stability, and on the mental and physical health of the teenagers and their children. In summary, prevention activities in CMHCs in the next decade will focus on smaller, higher-risk populations—particularly those with relevance for CMHC clinical caseloads.

Reduced funding and increased demands for services have fueled an increased emphasis on accountability among policymakers and funding sources. Prevention programs are expected to demonstrate scientific rigor and document positive outcomes to qualify for consideration in today's competitive arena of human services. The field of prevention of mental illness is a relative newcomer to the scientific enterprise. Even so, over the last decade it has produced sufficient documentation to silence the critical query turned cliche: "How can you prove you've prevented something that doesn't happen?" There now exists a veritable compendium of studies that have applied the methodologies of social and in some cases the medical and biological sciences to the field of prevention (Kessler & Albee, 1977; Munoz, 1976; Task Panel on Prevention, 1978). The use of pre- and posttests and control groups embedded in classic experimental and quasi-experimental designs has produced solid prevention research. Readers seeking information about the theory and application of prevention methodologies are referred to Lorion (1983) and Price and Smith (1985). Another recent addition to the burgeoning documentation of the science of prevention is found in a special issue of the *American Journal of Community Psychology* (1982). After a two-year process in which 49 prevention research studies were considered, 9 studies were accepted for publication based on criteria that included scientific rigor and positive outcomes. Hermalin and Morell (1981) have also addressed evaluation issues in prevention, and present several concrete models in their review.

A critical issue underlying CMHC prevention planning is how decisions are made to allocate available resources to prevention. The decision-making process encompasses a variety of inter-dependent systems, including (a) the CMHC, itself; (b) agencies, businesses, and citizen groups within the local community; and (c) the layers of local and national government that set the laws and policies within which the CMHC operates. There are four major issues the prevention planner must confront at each systems level. The first relates to the priority of the prevention mission. The second has to do with the appropriate role of the planner within each system. The third issue is that of capturing adequate resources for prevention programming. The final issue involves building or accessing a constituency for prevention. Each issue will be discussed in turn.

THE COMMUNITY MENTAL HEALTH CENTER

The Priority of the Prevention Missions with the CMHC

The priority of the prevention mission is often articulated in the center's mission statement. In response to both federal priorities and local citizens' initiatives, many CMHCs incorporated prevention goals into their centers' mission statements during the 1970s. Although the data indicated that these goals were honored more in lip service than in practice (Snow & Swift, 1985), in many centers these mission statements are still operative. In these cases the prevention planner can use this evidence to advocate for strengthening the commitment of the CMHC board and administration to prevention goals.

The end of federal funding for CMHCs and the shift to block grants have significantly reduced what was an already minimal commitment of CMHC resources to prevention (Armstrong, 1985; Dowell & Ciarlo, 1983; Snow & Swift, 1985). Traditionally, consultation and education units within CMHCs have been responsible for fulfilling the prevention function. In a five-year period in the 1970s, during the boom years of plentiful grant funding, no more than 5% of all CMHC staff hours went into consultation and education activities (Hassler, 1981). Only half of these hours, at best, were related to preventive programs (Vayda & Perlmutter, 1977). In sum, only 2.5% of all CMHC staff hours were devoted to prevention during the era when federal funds supported this function.

In the 1980s CMHCs are free from having to fulfill the regulations that dictated the allocation of resources in the 1960s and 1970s. Instead of having to provide 13 separate mental health services to residents in their catchment areas, CMHCs can now choose which services to provide based on the community's needs, and its economic and political realities. The consequences of this change for prevention programming within CMHCs have been largely negative. Since the end of federal funding for CMHCs, prevention programming has declined from a precariously supported service to an almost invisible one (Abt

Associates, 1976; Armstrong, 1985; Naierman, Haskins, & Robinson, 1978; Weiner et al., 1979). In most CMHCs the consultation and education unit has either been significantly reduced or dismantled entirely.

For some CMHC preventionists, then, securing a high priority—or any priority at all—for prevention services within the CMHC in the 1980s is a holding action aimed more at avoiding erosion of status than claiming a larger share of the center's resources.

The Role of the Prevention Planner Within the CMHC

Within the center the planner should make prevention goals and services highly visible. One way to do this is to establish a unit or program area with the word "prevention" in its title. The CMHC may provide an array of preventive services categorized under other labels. For example, early intervention programs targeted to high-risk mothers and children may be part of the center's official "Children's Services." Proactive programs with senior citizens may fall under the center's "Services for the Elderly." Prevention services gain legitimacy with recognition of their relevance to the center's comprehensive service system and its priority populations. The prevention planner should seek to group all of the CMHC's preventive services within a single prevention unit, and to head this unit as manager or director. Whatever the title, it is important that the prevention planner be a member of the center's administrative team. This assures participation in decisions that affect future center directions and allocation of resources. Optimum staffing for the prevention unit would provide a combination of full- and half-time positions. If the resources for this are lacking, designating specific CMHC staff with a percentage of their time allocated to prevention maintains the planner's authority and flexibility in assigning staff resources. Negotiating for both program staff and other CMHC resources—such as clerical support, computer access, equipment, and office space—is a fundamental part of the role of the prevention planner. Advocating for preventive services with the

CMHC's citizen board, administration, and staff is also a significant part of the planner's internal role.

Sources of CMHC Funding for Prevention Programs

There are three major types of funding for CMHC prevention programs: fees for services, mainstream CMHC funds, and grants. Generating fees to cover the costs of preventive services has been a low yield activity. The average annual dollar amount of fees generated in CMHC by consultation and education services did not exceed $11,000 per center across the years of federal support. This amount is less than 1% of total CMHC receipts from all revenue sources (Hassler, 1980). This record reflects, in part, the minimal investment of resources in the prevention function, differing models of fee recovery for preventive versus treatment services, and a lack of expertise in the prevention field in general, and CMHCs in particular, in delivering preventive services during that period (Dowell & Ciarlo, 1983).

Although fee-for-service mechanisms such as direct client billing and third party reimbursement were built into CMHC clinical treatment programs from the beginning, there is no comparable practice of fee collection for CMHC prevention programming. The failure to build fee-for-service strategies for prevention is rooted in both ideology and logistics. Ideologically, the official CMHC philosophy has been that prevention activities benefit the community at large. Because everyone has an investment in preventing mental illness, "everyone" pays for it through taxes. In practice, this means no one pays for it on an individual basis.

Logistically, the funding difficulty revolves around two dilemmas. One has to do with the inability to identify those who benefit from preventive services, and the other with the temporal contingencies involved. It is impossible to predict with certainty which individuals out of a given population at risk will benefit from preventive interventions. If an intervention succeeds in reducing the incidence of disorder in a population, it is clear that a proportion of the population has been spared or "saved" from the disorder. But it is impossible, in general, to identify which individual members would have been afflicted in the absence of the intervention. Because those persons "saved" by the preventive effort cannot be billed, in effect the entire community ends up paying.

CMHC treatment and preventive services both focus on the same outcome. Both are directed to eliminating mental illness. Neither service has an unequivocal record of success. However, payment for treatment services follows each treatment session, regardless of the effectiveness of the session. This is the familiar fee-for-service medical model. Prevention services, on the other hand, apply to well persons, not to DSM-diagnosed persons or the "worried well." Healthy individuals are asked to pay to stay that way. Payment is demanded "up front," prior to an event, to ward off the event. In general, efforts at such before-the-fact fee collection have been unsuccessful. However, when a disease or health threat reaches a critical incidence level, or a level of damage or disruption that constitutes an unacceptable threat to the quality of life or stability of the community, the likelihood increases that funds will be found to prevent the disorder.

A look at the few prevention programs that have gained community support demonstrates the point. When behaviors such as alcoholism, drug abuse, child abuse, and spouse abuse are perceived as sufficiently disruptive to a community, resources are then allocated to prevent these special problems. In general, disorders that compel such community response are those that affect a large number of people, or those that result in major suffering, incapacity, or disruption for the person directly affected, their families, coworkers, and other associates.

Community response to Acquired Immune Deficiency Syndrome (AIDS) is an example. Some public resources have gone into a search for a vaccine to prevent the disease, but the magnitude of these resources has been increasing as the disease spreads from a narrow set of populations at risk (male homosexuals, drug addicts, those receiving blood transfusions, and Haitians) to the broader community. AIDS now threatens the population at large (increasing incidence). In addition, the prognosis for those afflicted is extremely negative: With current treatment methods, death is a certain outcome within a few years of diagnosis. The magnitude of the resulting devastation for victims, their families, and the larger community is leading and will continue to lead to larger and larger commitments of resources to prevention efforts. The lesson here for CMHC preventionists is that fees for prevention services are most likely to be captured when the conditions to be prevented have "target relevance" for the community (Rich & Goldsmith, 1983).

CMHC mainstream funds are a second source of potential support. These are unrestricted funds that accrue to the center— through city and county tax levies and some state funds. It is the prevention planner's role to advocate for a share of these funds to be allocated to preventive programs. As noted above, to do this most effectively the planner should be a member of the administrative team. One rationale supporting "inside" lobbying is that consultation and education services are, collectively, one of the five services required for CMHCs to be eligible for federal block grant funds.

The Alcohol, Drug Abuse and Mental Health (ADM) Services Block Grant requires that consultation and education services be provided by centers as a condition of funding. "The regulations give the states maximum flexibility and discretion—and provide for minimal reporting burdens.... Although C & E is one of the required services under the ADM Block Grant, contact with state mental health officials indicates general concurrence with CMHC staff concerns that C & E will receive lower priority among the mandated services" (Stockdill, 1982, p. 22). Because there are no federal guidelines specifying what proportion of the funds should go to consultation and education, centers are bound only by state regulations in allocating scarce federal dollars between these services and clinical services.

In the absence of guidelines it is difficult for the planner to calculate what proportion of mainstream funds to request for prevention programs. Based on the record, and in the context of competing demands for clinical services, a figure of 5% of the center's total budget is a reasonable starting point for negotiations with the center director. The planner should be prepared to present a budget broken out by program areas justifying the amount requested. Clearly, CMHC prevention programs in the 1980s are not adequately supported by either fees or mainstream CMHC funds. The prevention planner will need to seek grants from both the public and private sectors to carry out even a modest level of programming.

Building a Constituency for Prevention Within the CMHC

The importance of building a constituency for prevention cannot be overemphasized (Cooper, 1980; Tableman, 1984). There should be support from within the CMHC, the local community, and at the state and national levels. Within the CMHC itself, the support of the board and the center director are critical. As noted above, board commitment is reflected in the center's mission statement and in the establishment of priorities for services. The planner should see to it through periodic presentations and reports to the board, articles in newsletters, and bulletins that board members are informed of prevention activities. In addition, the results of preventive interventions should appear in the center's annual reports and evaluations.

The current reality is that even with the ideological support of the CMHC board and director, it may be difficult to capture a significant share of center resources for prevention efforts. Saul Cooper, a 25-year prevention veteran of the community mental health movement, brings his experience as a CMHC director to an analysis of the barriers to prevention programming within CMHCs: "When typical administrators find themselves in the normative situation of having insufficient resources to meet already identified demands, they are most reluctant to look at other needs which may exist in the community. This needs-versus-demands issue is especially critical for those agencies interested in implementing prevention programs. It is almost as if clinical demands which are readily visible and which reflect the communities' press on the agency must be balanced against long-term prevention promises. In such a formula, clinical demands will almost always win'' (Cooper, 1980, p. 256). This is a clear message to the prevention planner that maintaining a CMHC base during economic austerity means focusing resources on populations already prominent on the center's clinical caseloads.

In the current economic climate, then, a strong case can be made that the initial focus for constituency building for prevention should be among members of populations with highly visible, demonstrated mental health needs, and with the organizations and agencies who serve them. The chronically mentally ill are at the top of this list. Children and elderly, minorities, and the poor are populations with ''target relevance'' for both treatment and prevention services. These groups all have their own constituencies advocating for increased services. Alliance with these groups can lead to the identification of common goals, collaborative programming, and a network of community support.

THE LOCAL COMMUNITY

The Priority of the Prevention Mission Within the Local Community

Assessing the priority of the prevention mission within local communities involves identifying persons, organizations, and agencies already doing prevention work. Although CMHC preventionists can directly affect the prevention priority within CMHCs, they have no insider's advantage in moving the prevention agenda through other community agencies and institutions. The task here is to seek support through constituency building and collaborative programming. The first step is to identify prevention peers within the community.

One barometer of the community's prevention priorities can be seen in the ways in which it deals with its vulnerable populations, such as children, minorities, the elderly, and the poor. Agencies promoting the welfare of children often house prevention projects. Early intervention programs are supported by public institutions such as health and welfare departments and departments of education, as well as by private hospitals, child guidance clinics, and mental health centers. Pregnant women are targeted for a wide range of preventive interventions, with special attention to high-risk groups such as teenagers and single, poor, and minority women. Agencies and groups involved in this work, in addition to those mentioned above, include La Leche League, Lamaze, and a variety of church groups.

The self-help movement has become a major force in prevention practice in the last decade (Borman, Borck, Hess, & Pasquale, 1982). In most U.S. communities there are active groups covering a wide range of situations, conditions, and problems. A project taken on by many CMHC preventionists in recent years is the publication of a resource and referral manual listing the self-help groups in the local community. Producing and disseminating the manual to local agencies and human service providers benefits the CMHC prevention program in several ways. It brings visibility to the CMHC and its prevention unit, establishes links between the CMHC and individual self-help groups, and casts the CMHC in a leadership role in organizing community resources.

The Role of the CMHC Prevention Planner in the Community

There are multiple tasks associated with the planner's public role. Basic to all other tasks is the assessment of community needs and resources. A second function is to serve as the CMHC's prevention representative to the community; this involves public education and consultation around prevention issues (Snow & Swift, 1985). A third function is that of information and referral for prevention services. In addition, advocating for prevention with community agencies and groups is an integral part of the role.

Of these tasks, the only one directly linked to the planning process is the assessment of community needs and resources. A program that makes sound prevention sense in one community may be a waste of resources in another. Programs directed to preventing the accumulation of toxic levels of lead in children illustrate the point. When these programs are implemented in an inner city metropolis, they meet scientific, logistical, and political criteria for effective preventive interventions. The scientific community has established the damage to health and mental health that results when children eat lead-based paint, or breathe toxic levels of lead pollutants from traffic emissions. Removing paint and reducing lead pollutants are tasks within the capacities of most cities to do. By supporting these programs local governments can demonstrate responsiveness to the needs of several important constituencies at once. The focus on safeguarding children's health is popular and safe. Mobilizing human resources to accomplish the task creates jobs. In the process, the environment is improved not just for children but for the entire community. On the other hand, this prevention program would be a waste of time and money in most suburbs, where neither residual paint nor traffic levels warrant concern. Targeting programs to community needs requires knowledge of its demography, ecology, economy, politics, and history. A comprehensive needs assessment can provide this information.

There are two important outcomes of a community needs assessment: the information it produces, and the process of constituency building and community education it generates. Basic information produced by the assessment includes general population statistics such as age, sex, race, income, education, and occupation, and a detailed analysis of the social and economic characteristics of the population served. Ideally this information should be available for each neighborhood. In this way the community's major population clusters can be located. The planner also needs to know which populations in the community are at high risk for developing mental health disorders and where these populations are located.

Familiarity with the history of a community assists the planner in understanding its values and traditions. This knowledge sheds light on community response to issues such as school busing, daycare, and comparable worth. Traditional attitudes valuing autonomy, for example, may impede help-seeking behavior, making interventions involving self-help groups problematic. The businesses and industries that form a community's economic base may carry hazards for employees, their families, or the community at large. A chemical plant or nuclear power plant has potential impact on both the physical and mental health of surrounding residents, particularly if there has been a history of insensitive or careless management. Communication and transportation networks have a daily impact on vital transactions within a community, such as accessibility to jobs, health care, and other services. The economic health of a community is reflected in a variety of mental health indices. Child abuse, spouse abuse, alcoholism, and depression have been directly linked to unemployment (Buss & Redburn, 1983).

Because few CMHC prevention planners in the 1980s will command sufficient center resources to conduct large-scale needs assessments, the planner will need to draw heavily on existing records and reports. Two major sources are archival records—in the form of CMHC grant applications and reports to federal agencies—and the Health Demographic Profile System—available through the National Institute of Mental Health (NIMH).

Prior to 1980, federally funded CMHCs were required to assess their community's needs and resources as a condition of funding. These assessments may now need to be updated, but they provide a beginning information base for program planning. The community's history, geography and a description of its economic base (major businesses, industries, agricultural products, and so on) can be found in the narrative of proposals for staffing and construction grants. This material, which became standard "boiler plate" in applications—was routinely updated with each new grant submission. Retrieving the first and last accounts of these community descriptions provides a brief but adequate historical perspective, and is likely to yield valuable sociological information as well.

During the 1970s NIMH required each federally funded CMHC to submit an annual inventory providing data on the community's utilization of center services. In addition, many grants required periodic progress reports. These reports now serve as expert sources of information for the prevention planner. Data for the CMHC prevention component—consultation and education services—were reported on the annual inventory as the number of staff hours per month delivered to specific populations. These populations were as follows: children, the general public, state and local law enforcement agencies, health services, substance abuse providers and their clients, other mental health agencies, public welfare agencies and their clients, the elderly, and other.

In addition, centers that have management information systems in place have the capacity to provide detailed information on consultation and education programs and individual staff contacts with the agencies and populations cited. Knowing the background of the CMHC's relationship with the community's schools or law enforcement agencies, for example, may guide the planner in building collaborative relationships or designing interventions. The annual inventories and reports described here should be a part of each center's archives.

The Health Demographic Profile System (HDPS), formerly known as the Mental Health Demographic Profile System (MHDPS), is an extremely useful set of data made up of social and economic indicators based on the 1980 U.S. census. The system can be used to analyze, describe, and compare populations, conduct needs assessment and service-utilization studies, locate risk populations within communities, and project incidence and prevalence rates for a variety of physical and mental illnesses (Goldsmith, Jackson, Doenhoefer, & Johnson, 1984). The original system (MHDPS), based on the 1970 census, provided 131 social and economic indicators. The revised set of HDPS indicators is organized into seven broad categories: General Population Data (general, rural/urban); Ethnic Composition; Socioeconomic Status (income, poverty or welfare populations, house value, rent value, employment level and labor force participation, social status, educational status); Household Composition and Family Structure (general characteristics, marital status, family life cycle—including families with children, families with female householder, mothers in the labor force, young families, early or middle childbearing families, older households, and persons not in families); Housing Characteristics (type of housing, condition of housing, overcrowding); Residential Mobility; and Disabled Population. The data currently exist on computer tapes at NIMH in the form of raw numbers, percentages, medians, and quartiles. The system has the capacity to retrieve these data by geographic areas as small as blocks and as large as the nation.

The system is based on the prevention premise that disorders are not randomly distributed in a population. Disorders have been found to cluster in certain neighborhoods, age groups, or economic classes. Persons in such clusters are labeled "at risk." In general, persons are considered to be at risk if they are members of a group in which the incidence of a specified disorder is above the base rate for that disorder in the population (Vance, 1977). Poverty is a risk factor, as is divorce, frequent geographic moves, and under- or unemployment. Patterns of socioeconomic indicators have been associated with infant mortality, poverty, segregation, alcoholism, suicide, personal disorganization, delinquency, retardation, and mental illness (Redick, Goldsmith, & Unger, 1971).

In addition to standard demographic data, HDPS has a special set of indicators developed to identify populations at high risk for developing mental disorders. Examples of such populations at risk are teenagers not in school, aged persons living alone, divorced or separated males and females, and female-headed families with children in poverty. A set of indicators has also been developed for three special target populations: children, women, and the elderly. By utilizing HDPS data for their local communities, prevention planners can produce a quick, highly sophisticated needs assessment. Such HDPS data, in combination with data documenting the utilization of center services by various populations, are also useful in identifying gaps in service delivery and unserved or underserved populations.

In the 1970s MHDPS data in the form of computer printouts were routinely made available to all state mental health authorities and to individuals on request. With the advent of block grants and the elimination of the NIMH's technical assistance function, these data are more difficult to obtain, although still available. Now, instead of printouts, HDPS data are distributed in the form of computer tapes. The set of HDPS data for each state is being sent only to state mental health authorities on request, however. Individuals must access the data through their state authority.

Another needs assessment technique, the community forum, is a scaled down version of the old town meeting. Citizens with a special interest in a topic of importance to the community meet to hear formal presentations from "experts," then discuss and vote their opinions. A third needs assessment technique, noted for yielding a large volume of information relative to the small group of citizens involved, is the nominal group. This method involves a highly structured group exercise in which participants generate responses to questions about the community's problems and possible solutions. Detailed instructions on how to implement these techniques can be found in Hagedorn et al. (1976). As valuable as the information provided is the constituency building accomplished by needs assessment techniques that bring members of the community together to consider issues bearing on their welfare. If the appropriate mix of invested citizens is brought together, the results can include not only information about the community's needs but the formation of an advocacy group committed to securing resources for a particular preventive program or policy.

Sources of Prevention Funding, and Constituency Building Within the Local Community

Building a constituency and developing program support within the community go hand in hand. Therefore, the two topics are combined for discussion here. The end of federal funding has forced CMHCs to appeal directly to their local communities for support. As part of an effort to market mental health services more aggressively and to package services more attractively, many centers have changed their names. Some have dropped the "mental health" label for the more encompassing and less stigmatizing "health center" label. Others have incorporated trendier words such as "growth" or "holistic" into their corporate identities. Along with shifts in center names has come relabeling of center services. Consultation and education services are now called "prevention services," or, more commonly, "consultation, education, and prevention" (CEP) services.

Currently, the most likely sources of fee income for prevention programs in the community are schools, businesses, and human service organizations, including health and mental health agencies. During the 1970s, schools were the major source of fee income for consultation, education, and prevention services. CMHCs that had received federal funds the longest during that period—from 6-7 years of federally supported operations—derived over half of their consultation and education fees from schools. This compares with no school dollars for CMHCs in their first few years of operation, or in the years following their graduation from federal support—8-9 years after startup (Hassler, 1980). The consultation and education interventions that earned reimbursement from schools were case and program consultation and staff training. Case consultation in schools is primarily a clinical service, but it also serves prevention goals. It assists teachers in resolving particular cases, and increases the teachers' expertise in recognizing and preventing similar cases in the future. Reductions in local and federal funding have affected schools and CMHCs simultaneously. Faced with survival, schools in the 1980s have quit paying for consultation, training, and other preventive services, and many CMHCs have quit offering them.

It is unlikely, in view of the current crisis in funding in education, that schools will be able to pay for preventive services from regularly budgeted funds. However, some of the leading "success models" in the field of prevention involve schools as sites and children as target populations (Alpert & Associates, 1982; Gesten & Weissberg, 1982; Shure & Spivack, 1982). Prevention planners seeking funding to replicate these models are advised to approach local sources—foundations and businesses. If the planner has attended to the process of building a prevention constituency and community consensus around program priorities, citizen leaders will make the case for funding preventive interventions in schools (Tableman, 1984).

Businesses and industries in a community influence the prevention planning process primarily through the direct purchase of preventive services for their employees. They also provide program funding through contributions and corporate gifts. Finally, they influence the process through their advocacy for prevention in civic circles where the community's corporate and political policymakers are found.

Increasingly, businesses are eliciting the assistance of mental health consultants in designing employee assistance programs (EAPs) and benefit packages responsive to the complex problems and multiple lifestyles represented in today's worksite. EAPs generally package a variety of preventive interventions and clinical services, with the aim of increasing productivity and reducing inefficiency, accidents, and absenteeism at work. A common preventive strategy is educating employees about issues of health and mental health. Stress management, smoking cessation, promotion of nutrition, and exercise are standard parts of an EAP package. Management consultation and supervisor training are additional EAP components with preventive potential. Consulting with management around substantive programs and personnel issues and policies such as flex time, shared jobs, health benefits, and vacations has clear preventive implications. Training supervisors to recognize staff burnout, signs of risk for addictive disorders such as alcohol or drug abuse, or other mental health problems, and educating supervisors in community resources and referral networks is also good prevention work.

How successful have EAPs proved to be in generating fee income for CMHCs? In a recent survey of mental health agencies, 42% of the respondents listed consultation to private industry as a source of fee income (Backer et al., 1983). However, the median annual income reported for EAPs by respondents is $10,000; the average income generated is $36,663. These figures include income for both clinical and consultation and education services. From these figures, it appears that EAPs have not proved to be a major revenue stream for preventive services to date.

A potentially lucrative source of funds from the private sector lies in the broad field of staff development and training. Many businesses and industries maintain an in-house training staff, and many firms budget funds for employees to receive outside training. The substantive content of the training varies widely, with the industry and the needs of particular employees. Some firms contract with colleges and universities to reserve slots in selected classes for their employees. Others bring in outside consultants or trainers for educational events at the worksite. CMHCs have had little contact with these programs. Planners wishing to explore possible preventive agendas within this field are advised to review journals such as that published by the Administrative Management Society and other professional training groups.

Cooper (1980) has suggested service clubs—such as Kiwanis, Rotary, and Junior League—and church groups as possible community bases for prevention programs. Special interest groups and small businesses can provide support in many ways. As members of other community organizations and boards, they wield political influence. If the goals of a particular prevention program are congruent with their interests, they may provide funds or in-kind services. Funeral directors have contributed to the development of self-help groups for the bereaved, for example, through grants, by referring clients to groups, and by distributing group literature. Local printers sometimes print brochures or newsletters free of charge. Local outlets of national chains may support community causes as a matter of policy or may develop on a local basis a program supported by their national office (e.g., Ronald McDonald houses for parents with hospitalized children).

Health and mental health organizations within a community are in key positions to influence preventive services both directly and indirectly. They exercise direct influence as providers and consumers of preventive services, and as gatekeepers in directing referrals. The indirect influence of these organizations is reflected in public policies as well as in the systems of reimbursement set up in the private sector to recover the costs of services.

It has become increasingly difficult, in the 1980s, to separate definitively the fields of health and mental health. The definition of health, according to the World Health Organization, is "a state of complete physical, mental and social well-being and is not merely the absence of disease and infirmity" (Albino, 1983). The CMHC preventionist must develop liaisons with health professionals and organizations in the home community as an integral part of prevention planning—both to avoid duplication of services and to coordinate referrals, contracts, and collaborative programming. With the advent of health maintenance organizations (HMOs), the preventive emphasis of health care has achieved new prominence. There are sound business reasons for this. By encouraging people to adopt healthy lifestyles and to take responsibility for their own well-being, health costs are reduced.

Health clinics and hospitals are major providers of preventive services, including health education, self-help groups, and early intervention programs. Topics of workshops and seminars offered to the public range from smoking cessation to nutrition and family planning. When these services cannot be provided in-house, hospitals contract with outside providers to supply them. Many CMHCs have formed alliances with their local hospitals and health clinics to present jointly or to subcontract health education offerings to the public.

Early intervention programs are a classic and well-tested prevention initiative, focusing on high-risk mothers and their children (Heber & Garber, 1975; Moss, Hess, & Swift, 1982). Most hospitals and clinics with obstetric units offer one or more components of an early intervention program, though few have the resources to provide follow-up care past the first year after birth. Responsibility for these programs can be distributed among a number of community agencies, including the local city and county health departments, the school system, the visiting nurses' association, and the local CMHC.

A third area of prevention programming for hospitals is in providing self-help groups for patients and their families. Most serious medical conditions are now represented in the ranks of the burgeoning self-help movement. For example, patients in most urban areas who are undergoing mastectomies, those with cancer, Alzheimer's disease, or multiple schlerosis can link themselves through self-help groups to others with similar conditions. Here again, if the local hospital lacks the resources to support such groups, the CMHC may work collaboratively with the hospital to provide them, or may offer self-help groups to supplement hospital services.

Health and mental health organizations are bidirectional gatekeepers in their control of service utilization. They control access to their own services and they direct those they serve to other agencies and services within the community. What this means for prevention planners is that they should establish and maintain active liaisons with representatives of other health and mental health agencies in their communities. If a network of prevention practitioners does not exist, it is advisable to build one. Networking may occur formally, through cosponsored events and contracted consultation. Or it may occur informally, through shared resources—such as staff and materials—such as audiovisual equipment, or access to target populations.

Hospitals and clinics also consume preventive services through staff training. In the classic training of trainers model, preventionists train community gatekeepers in prevention techniques to improve their skills in processing people through society's basic institutions. Education, law enforcement, health care, and social services have been the primary institutions targeted. By consulting with and training teachers, police officers, physicians and nurses, and other human service workers in preventive methods, the populations served by these groups stand to gain in coping skills and social support. The prevention planner should set the fees for these services to make them self-supporting.

Increasingly, private foundations are committing resources to prevention initiatives. However, many foundations do not recognize these initiatives as relating to mental health, and thus are not inclined to fund CMHC prevention programs. Areas of interest for private foundations today include daycare, respite care for families caring for elders or disabled family members in their homes, and research and policy support for flex time, job sharing, and revisions of health and benefits packages at the worksite to reflect changing roles in the family. The CMHC planner seeking private funds for such prevention programs may be in the position of having to translate them into mental health terms for both the CMHC administrator and foundation officials.

GOVERNMENT: LOCAL, STATE, AND FEDERAL

The Priority of the Prevention Mission Within the Local, State, and Federal Governments

Each community has a unique political and economic context that shapes the social service delivery system. Examples include the recession and rebound of the automobile industry in Detroit, the continuing depression of communities whose economies are based on steel or coal, and the boom of high-tech industries in Silicon Valley, Boston, and the North Carolina Triangle. It is the business of the prevention planner to be familiar with the unique conditions that shape the local economy and government.

In the 1980s, economic forces common to all U.S. communities have forged a political consensus within local governments around essential and nonessential services in general, and prevention services in particular. Pressed by the urgent needs of populations such as the chronically mentally ill, the poor, and the homeless, local governments are without the resources to support the broad goal of preventing mental illness in the general population. Rich and Goldsmith (1983) recently surveyed a group of policymakers—legislators, mental health officials, service providers, and advocacy groups—about their priorities for mental health services. They found that state and local policymakers support the concept of prevention but give it a relatively low priority for funding. Respondents ranked preventive services below services for underserved populations— such as youth, the elderly, and the chronically mentally ill— and below the fiscal goals of accountability, reimbursements, and reform of Medicare/Medicaid and other third-party payers.

In view of the state of economic siege that human services currently find themselves in, these priorities are understandable. Rich and Goldsmith suggest three reasons for the consistent but relatively weak support for prevention reflected in survey results. First, policymakers are not convinced that prevention programs can be measured. Second, it is unclear how prevention programs can be held fiscally accountable. Third, there are no clear guidelines for deciding how to allocate scarce resources between the amorphous goal of prevention and the specific needs of the chronically mentally ill.

Because of the fuzziness of prevention goals and methodologies in the eyes of local policymakers, in contrast with the specific rankings of underserved populations, they see few options to committing available funds to the poor, the elderly, and the chronically mentally ill. In order to make a credible case for funding prevention in this decade, the target populations must be relevant to the populations that burden the larger social service system—a theme echoed throughout this chapter. Children of the chronically mentally ill, for example, are at higher risk for developing disorders than other children (Goodman, 1984). Interventions with this population can serve both prevention and treatment goals. Such interventions can reduce the incidence of disorder in the children, and at the same time contribute to the adjustment of the chronically mentally ill parent. As Rich and Goldsmith point out, there must be a clear connection between the at-risk caseloads of prevention programs and the caseloads clogging the mental health service system:

> "target-relevance" will have a strong influence on resource allocations. To the extent that prevention is perceived as a phenomenon to be applied generically, to the populations at large,

it will remain outside the mainstream of mental health policy-making. Conversely, to the extent that the prevention community can demonstrate "clinically-related" effectiveness for specific target groups of high priority to policymakers, prevention may become incorporated into that "mainstream" (as represented by funding appropriations and allocations). (Rich & Goldsmith, 1983, p. 21)

Today, local and state governments are the dominating influence that shape CMHC prevention programs. Cities provide the citizen volunteers who staff advisory groups and boards, the consumers who utilize mental health services, the leaders who establish community priorities, and the network of human service agencies whose mandates and services overlap and cross those of the CMHC. Counties may provide these resources as well, but they also contribute funds through the exercise of mill levies and other taxes. In the 1980s, state government has adopted the role formerly played by the federal government in overseeing the operations of CMHCs.

The prevention of mental illness currently enjoys its highest federal priority in history at the level of policy. It is paradoxical that this elevated status comes at a time when federal dollars for CMHC prevention programs have been severely reduced. The few NIMH prevention funds that are available are being channeled into research. Since President John Kennedy first articulated prevention goals in the first Presidential Message on Mental Health, the concept has gained support through multiple levels of government.

At the federal level of government alone, a conservative count of agencies with responsibilities or functions related to prevention shows 11 departments, 17 independent agencies, 3 quasi-official agencies, 5 permanent or temporary offices within the Executive Office of the President, and 4 agencies within the legislative branch. This count does not include Congressional committees and subcommittees with jurisdiction of health- or prevention-related areas. In fact, most preventive activities at the federal level lie outside the Department of Health, Education and Welfare, especially those that involve regulatory or enforcement authority. Such activities include food and nutrition programs administered by the Department of Agriculture, occupational health and safety programs administered by the Department of Labor, environmental control programs administered by the Environmental Protection Agency and other agencies, and most consumer product safety programs. (Franks, 1981, pp. 1-2)

Federal support for prevention has been written into legislation, as seen in section 455 of the Public Health Services Act (PL 96-398, 1982), and codified in departments and positions within the federal bureaucracy. Some of the institutional changes and some sources of financial support for the prevention of mental illness are reviewed below.

The Role of the Prevention Planner Vis-à-Vis Local, State, and Federal Government

The broad role of the CMHC preventionists vis à vis governmental agencies involved three primary tasks: to engage in information exchange, resource development, and advocacy for legislation and policies promoting prevention. Information exchange involves maintaining a continuous stream of current information from each level of government, and seeing to it that key officials receive updated reports about CMHC prevention programs. Standard sources of information include local newspapers, the Federal Register, and bulletins and requests for proposals (RFPs) from local, state, and federal agencies. National newsletters with specific prevention information include the *Prevention Quarterly* of the National Council of Community Mental Health Centers; the *Division 27 Newsletter* published by the Division of Community Psychology of the American Psychological Association; *Idea Interchange,* published by the NIMH Mental Health Education Branch; and newsletters of professional associations such as the American Psychiatric Association, the National Association of Social Workers, and the American Sociological Association. Through active resource development, the preventionist is informed of current RFPs and grant initiatives from the various public agencies.

One of the major roles of state and federal governments is to formulate and implement public policy. "Once an issue. . . becomes labeled a social problem, it inevitably becomes linked with public policy. This fact implies that any solutions will then be based on compromise regarding values and political constituencies as much as on scientific findings from any discipline" (Repucci, Mulvey, & Kastner, 1983). Public policy is an area in which few prevention professionals have become involved. The consequences of this default position is that preventionists now have to live with health and mental health policies that were developed without their input and that, in many cases, are inimical to their interests (Keisler, 1980). As Sarason (1983, p. 246) notes, "Any individual or field that purports to be interested in understanding and/or influencing the dynamics of our communities has to become sophisticated about public policy."

The entire fee structure for reimbursing mental health services, the priorities that put treatment of the chronically mentally ill ahead of preventive programs, the delivery of control over prevention programs into the hands of those unsympathetic to its ideology—these are some of the results of the failure of prevention professionals to make their voices heard at the level of policymaking during the 1960s and 1970s. Public policy decisions at the federal level that most directly affect CMHC prevention programs are made by the Department of Health and Human Services, and implemented through the prevention offices of NIMH, the National Institute on Alcohol Abuse and Alcoholism, and the National Institute on Drug Abuse.

Tableman (1984) investigated state prevention programs through a survey of state departments of mental health. She found 17 states that sponsor preventive activities, with resources ranging from $16,000 (New Hampshire) to $1.3 million (Michigan). The diversity of state prevention programs is reflected in the administrative unit which this activity is housed within the State Department of Mental Health. In 4 states, prevention services are found within the federal block grant for substance abuse. Other administrative bases for prevention include children's services, training and education, research and development, and the executive office of the Department of Mental Health.

Based on the survey and her own experience as director of prevention programs for the State of Michigan, Tableman (1984) has formulated "axioms for the politics of the possible." They stress the uniqueness of each state in shaping programs to match state needs, the necessity to build a constituency for prevention, and the importance of translating broad visionary prevention goals into specific, cost-effective interventions targeted to at-risk populations that are relevant to the CMHC's clinical caseloads. Tableman (1984, p. 12) suggests that relevance, in this context, refers to a continuum of mental health services in which "the prevention caseload is the treatment caseload at an earlier point in time." She warns practitioners that unless prevention is defined in specific terms, and demonstrated to be cost effective, little support can be expected from state authorities:

> Legislators tend to be concrete thinkers. They can deal with specific populations and specific problems, but they have difficulty understanding what exactly is subsumed under preventing mental illness or such broad concepts as empowering people.... Whenever possible, plans, position papers or legislative poposals should specify: what you are proposing to prevent, what population you propose to serve, what you propose to do and the documentation from the risk factors and intervention literature that says this is a reasonable thing to do. (Tableman, 1984, p. 10)

Robert Okin (1977), when he was Commissioner of Mental Health for the State of Vermont, noted the difficulties that deter state officials from advocating for prevention programs. First, the overwhelming demands for services to those diagnosed with mental illness drain available resources. Whereas there are strong constituencies pushing for treatment services for alcohol and drug abusers and the chronically mentally ill, there are no groups that make a compelling case for preventive services. A secondary difficulty lies in the fact that many effective prevention programs are outside the jurisdiction of the mental health commissioner—such as daycare, planned parenthood, and income maintenance. A commissioner who fights for a mental health share of a small pool of state funds may be in the position of gaining money for treatment at the expense of excellent primary prevention programs operated by other state authorities:

> The ironic result is that the commissioner of mental health, though a sincere advocate of the need for primary prevention, often finds himself fighting against it through his actions. We are left with the paradox that a person who by virtue of this position could do a great deal to advance the cause of primary prevention can unwittingly become one of its foremost opponents. (Okin, 1977, p. 295)

There are several lessons here for the CMHC prevention planner. Much of the programming that is effective in preventing mental illness is initiated and maintained outside the official mental health system. The planner should be knowledgeable about the legislation, policies, funding initiatives, and key personnel that determine prevention's fortunes at every level of government.

Sources of Government Funding for CMHC Prevention Program

Public funds in the form of grants are currently a primary source of funding for CMHC prevention programs. An array of federal block grant monies are channeled through state governments. Some states earmark specific funds for favored programs. For example, in 1984 Massachusetts set aside $1 million for the prevention of sexual child abuse.

During the 1970s support for CMHC prevention programs was scattered across a broad range of federal agencies. The Department of Health, Education and Welfare (now HHS) encompassed a range of ideologies and funding mechanisms related to prevention within its institutes. Staffing and operations grants, consultation and education grants, and Part F Children's grants were the official NIMH mechanisms designed to fund preventive activities in CMHCs. Additional monies were available through the prevention offices of NIDA and NIAAA.

In the 1980s the federal domain of prevention in mental health has been organized and focused within NIMH. CMHC preventive services are no longer fundable per se. Research is now the priority for NIMH prevention dollars. Responsibility for prevention is divided into two units: the Office of Prevention and the Center for Prevention Research. These are the NIMH offices with which the CMHC prevention planner should be in contact. The planner should be listed to receive all new prevention grant initiatives as soon as they are released to the field, as well as annual reports and publication series of the Office of Prevention and initial and final reports of prevention research funded.

An Office of Prevention within the Office of the NIMH Director coordinates and develops policies, priorities, programs, and workshops; maintains liaison with other governmental and private agencies working in the area of prevention; and directs current research and related program developments to citizens and policymakers as an aid for policy and action alternatives. The Center for Prevention Research was created in 1982 within the Division of Special Mental Health Programs at NIMH. This center invites applications from the field for a variety of research initiatives.

The Division of Prevention within NIAAA has two branches: the Prevention Policy Branch and the Prevention Services Branch. NIAAA initially funded demonstration grants focusing on community prevention and youth education programs. Youth demonstration grants funded include the following: "school-based programs dealing with curriculum implementation, teacher training and peer training; strategies targeted toward school dropouts, runaways and street youth; programs designed by voluntary organizations to reach their memberships through nontraditional approaches; prevention strategies suitable for implementation on college campuses; and projects designed to train youth outreach workers in the early recognition of alcohol problems among youth" (ADAMHA, 1981).

NIAAA's (1981, p. 43) community demonstration grant program has funded a variety of prevention programs: "community organization techniques; approaches for Indian communities; a training program for black community gatekeepers; an alcohol training model for families; and a community intervention model." NIAAA has developed sets of training/education materials for prevention courses targeted at women, blacks, and parents of young children. Current emphases of NIAAA prevention demonstration grants include the ecology of drinking behavior—alcohol and combined media-community intervention approaches. In addition, in the 1970s NIAAA funded a staff position for prevention in 48 states. When this funding ended in 1977, 47 states continued to fund these positions.

NIDA is the only federal agency that had a portion of its budget mandated by Congress to be spent on drug abuse prevention and intervention activities. NIDA's dedicated funding began in 1980 with 7% and was increased in 1981 to 10%. Beginning in 1983, NIDA prevention dollars were channeled through the block grant mechanism to the states, with 20% of the alcohol and drug portion set aside for prevention initiatives. NIDA's Prevention Branch supports a broad range of prevention strategies, including early and continuing education about the effects of drugs, decision-making processes and healthy development; interventions to alter the social climate of acceptability of drug use; and interventions that reduce individual and social stress factors.

A variety of other federal agencies also support prevention activities, although they may not always be so labeled. Prominent among these are agencies dealing with children, such as the Administration for Children, Youth and Families (ACYF), and the National Center for Child Abuse and Neglect (NCCAN). The Departments of Justice, Education, Labor and Housing and Urban Development all fund activities with clear preventive applications. By getting on the mailing lists of these agencies and reading government periodicals reporting their activities—such as the *Federal Register* and the *ADAMHA News*—the prevention planner can keep current on federal funding initiatives.

Building a National Constituency for Prevention

The CMHC prevention planner should have access to formal regional and national networks of peers. Many states and some regions have formed networks of CMHC prevention practitioners—although these have shrunk in the wake of funding cuts. The National Council of Community Mental Health Centers' Prevention Division provides members with a newsletter, an annual conference, and a network of CMHC prevention professionals on both the regional and national levels. This division has taken the lead in many national issues affecting prevention over the last decade. It has developed guidelines for consultation and education services (Snow & Swift, 1981). Together with the National Mental Health Association, the NCCMHC Prevention Division drafted the language for the prevention section of the Mental Health Systems Act.

The Vermont Conference on the Primary Prevention of Psychopathology (VCPPP), which meets annually at the University of Vermont in Burlington, is the site of a critical mass of prevention activity. The cutting edge of prevention scholarship and research is represented in the formal presentations and the informal conversations and networks that occur. For those unable to attend VCPPP, recommended reading is the set of published proceedings that document the work of the conference (Albee & Joffe, 1977-1984).

Both health and mental health organizations influence public policy through advocacy and lobbying for legislation and regulations favorable to their interests and through the support of political candidates sympathetic to their goals. Professional organizations such as the American Psychological Association, the National Association of Social Workers, and the National Council of Community Mental Health Centers alert their members to pending legislation (and regulations) affecting their interests. Members then respond by contacting local government officials and representatives to make their views clear and to recruit support for specific legislation. The advocacy of a constituency of professionals and the lay public for prevention achieved major advances in the Mental Health Systems Act, and in the currently operative Section 455 of the Public Services Act. The National Mental Health Association and their local chapters have played significant roles in advancing the cause of the prevention of mental illness. This organization's annual Lela Rowland Award contributes to strengthening prevention practice by recognizing exemplary prevention programs that have demonstrated effectiveness. The CMHC preventionist seeking a voice in the formulation of policy and a community of peers is invited to join one or more of these groups.

SUMMARY

This chapter reviews the process of prevention planning in community mental health centers from a systems perspective. The roles of various levels of the CMHC, the local community, and local and federal governments are outlined as they influence the planning process. Four basic issues that confront the planner are considered within the context of the CMHC, the local community and local, state, and federal governments: the priority of the prevention mission, the role of the prevention planner, sources of funding for CMHC prevention programs, and constituency building. It is argued that the appropriate goal of prevention activities in the 1980s is to reduce the incidence of specific disorders in at-risk populations that have relevance to CMHC clinical caseloads, using methods demonstrated to be effective. Because of the severe reduction in federal funds for human service programs, and the inability of the business world to fill this funding gap, CMHC prevention planners are challenged to develop innovative prevention programming using collaborative models that make maximum use of the resources of their CMHC setting and their local communities.

References

Abt Associates. (1976). *An evaluation of community mental health centers in their 10th and 11th years of operation.* Unpublished report. NIMH contract No. 100-76-0205.

ADAMHA prevention policy and programs, 1979-1982. (1981). DHHS Publication No. (ADM) 81-1038.

Albee, G., & Joffe, J. (General Eds.). (1977-1984). *The primary prevention of psychopathology* (Vols. I-VII). Hanover, NH: University Press of New England.

Albino, J. (1983). Health psychology and primary prevention: Natural allies. In R. Felner, L. Jason, J. Moritsugu, & S. Farber (Eds.), *Preventive psychology: Theory, research and practice,* (pp. 221-233). New York: Pergamon Press.

Alpert, J. (Ed.). (1982). *Psychological consultation in educational settings.* San Francisco: Jossey-Bass.

American Journal of Community Psychology. (1982). *10*(3).

Armstrong, D. (1985). *The graduation of consultation and education units of Massachusetts CMHCs from NIMH funding: Implications for the prevention mission of the community mental health center.* Doctoral dissertation, University of Massachusetts.

Backer, T., Shifren-Levine, I., & Erchul, W. (1983). *National survey of consultation and education programs.* Final report. Los Angeles: Human Interaction Research Institute.

Borman, L., Borck, L., Hess, R., & Pasquale, F. (Eds.). (1982). *Helping people to help themselves.* New York: Haworth Press.

Buss, T., & Redburn, F. (1983). *Mass unemployment.* Beverly Hills, CA: Sage.

Cooper, S. (1980). Implementing prevention programs: A community mental health center director's point of new. In R. Price, R. Ketterer, B. Bader, & J. Monahan (Eds.), *Prevention in mental health: Research policy and practice* (pp. 253-261). Beverly Hills, CA: Sage.

Dowell, D., & Ciarlo, J. (1983). Overview of the community mental health center's program from an evaluation perspective. *Community Mental Health Journal, 19*(2), 95-125.

Franks, P. (1981). Health policy and health planning: A framework for federal, state and local prevention initiative in the 1980s. In *The health care system and drug abuse prevention: Toward cooperation and health promotion.* DHHS Publication No. (ADS) 81-105, 1-12. Washington, DC: Government Printing Office.

Gesten, E. L., & Weissberg, R. P. (1982). Setting up and disseminating programs for social problem solving. In J. Alpert (Ed.), *Psychological consultation in educational settings* (pp. 208-246). San Francisco: Jossey-Bass.

Goldsmith, H., Jackson, D., Doenhoefer, S., & Johnson, W. (1984). *The health demographic profile system's inventory of small area social indicators.* DHHS Publication No. (ADM) 84-1354. Washington, DC: Government Printing Office.

Goodman, S. (1984). Children of disturbed parents: The interface between research and intervention. *American Journal of Community Psychology, 12*(6), 663-687.

Hagedorn, H., Beck, K., Neubert, S., & Werlin, S. (1976). *A working manual of simple program evaluation techniques for community mental health centers.* Stock No. 017-024-00539-8. Washington, DC: Government Printing Office.

Hassler, F. (1980). *Current national data and trends for C and E services.* Unpublished report. Staff College, National Institute of Mental Health, Rockville, MD.

Hassler, F. (1981). *Current national data and trends of C and E services.* Report prepared for the course "Developing and Managing Consultation and Education Services." Washington, DC: The Staff College, National Institute of Mental Health.

Heber, R., & Garber, H. (1975). The Milwaukee Project: A study of the use of family intervention to prevent cultural-familial mental retardation. In B. Friedlander, G. Sterritt, & G. Kirk (Eds.), *The exceptional infant: Assessment and intervention* (Vol. 3). New York: Brunner/Mazel.

Hermalin, J., & Morell, J. (1981). *Evaluation and prevention in human services.* New York: Haworth.

Keisler, C. (1980). Health Policy as a field of inquiry for psychology. *American Psychologist, 35,* 1066-1080.

Kessler, M., & Albee, G. (1977). An overview of the literature of primary prevention. In G. Albee, & J. Joffee (Eds.), *Primary prevention of psychopathology,* Vol. 1 (pp. 351-399). Hanover, NH: University Press of New England.

Lorion, R. (1983). Evaluating preventive interventions: Guidelines for the serious social change agent. In R. Felner, L. Jason, J. Moritsugu, & S. Farber (Eds.), *Preventive psychology theory, research and practice* (pp. 251-268) New York: Pergamon Press.

Moss, H., Hess, R., & Swift C. (Eds.). (1982). *Early intervention programs for infants.* New York: Haworth.

Munoz, R. (1976). The primary prevention of psychological problems. *Community Mental Health Review, 1*(6), 1-15.

Naierman, N., Haskins, B., & Robinson, G. (1978). *Community mental health centers—a decade later.* Cambridge, MA: Abt Associates.

Okin, R. (1977). Primary prevention of psychopathology from the perspective of a state mental health program director. In G. Albee & J. Joffe (Eds.), *Primary prevention of psychopathology.* (pp. 289-296). Hanover, NH: University Press of New England.

Price, R., & Smith, S. (1985). *A guide to evaluating prevention programs in mental health.* DHHS Publication No. (ADM) 85-1365. Washington, DC: Government Printing Office.

Redick, R., Goldsmith, H., & Unger, E. (1971). *1970 census data used to indicate areas with different potentials for mental health problems.* DHEW Publication No. (HSM) 73-9058. Washington, DC: Government Printing Office.

Reppucci, N., Mulvey, P., & Kastner, L. (1983). Prevention and interdisciplinary perspectives: A framework and case analysis. In R. Felner, L. Jason, J. Moritsugu, & S. Farber (Eds.), *Preventive psychology, theory, research and practice.* (pp. 234-244). New York: Pergamon Press.

Rich, R., & Goldsmith N. (1983). *Implementing Section 455 of the Public Health Service Law prevention and promotion of mental health.* Pittsburgh, PA: School of Urban Affairs, Carnegie-Mellon University.

Sarason, S. (1983). Psychology and public policy: Missed opportunity. In R. Felner, L. Jason, J. Moritsugu, & S. Farber (Eds.), *Preventive psychology, theory, research and practice.* (pp. 245-250). New York: Pergamon Press.

Shure, M., & Spivack G. (1982). Interpersonal problem solving in young children: A cognitive approach to prevention. *American Journal of Community Psychology, 10*(3), 341-356.

Snow, D., & Swift, C. (Eds.). (1981). *Recommended policies and procedures for consultation and education services within community mental health systems/agencies.* Washington, DC: National Council of Community Mental Health Center.

Snow, D., & Swift, C. (1985). Consultation and education in community mental health: A historical analysis. *The Journal of Primary Prevention 6*(1), 3-30.

Stockdill, J. (1982). ADM block grants: Political centers, implementation philosophy and issues related to consultation in mental health. *Consultation, 1,* 20-24.

Swift, C. (1980). Primary prevention, policy and practice. In R. Price, R. Ketterer, B. Bader, & J. Monahan (Eds.), *Prevention in mental health: Research, policy and practice.* (pp. 207-236). Beverly Hills, CA: Sage.

Tableman, B. (1984, June). *Statewide prevention programs: The politics of the possible.* Paper presented at the Tenth Annual Vermont Conference on Primary Prevention of Psychopathology, Burlington, VT.

Task Panel on Prevention. (1978). In *Report to the President from the President's Commission on Mental Health.* Washington, DC: Government Printing Office.

Vance, E. (1977). A typology of risks and the disabilities of low status. In G. Albee & J. Joffe (Eds.), *Primary prevention of psychopathology.* (pp. 207-237). Hanover, NH: University Press of New England.

Vayda, A. M., & Perlmutter, F. (1977). Primary prevention in community mental health centers: A survey of current activity. *Community Mental Health Journal 13,* 343-351.

Weiner, R., Woy, R., Sharfstein, S., & Bass, R. (1979). Community mental health centers and the 'seed money concept': Effects of terminating federal funds. *Community Mental Health Journal 15,* 129-138.

Chapter 5

PREVENTION PLANNING IN THE SCHOOL SYSTEM

JOEL MEYERS and RICHARD D. PARSONS

Professionals concerned with the prevention of mental health problems have always had a special interest in the potential preventive role to be played by the school system. Although prevention in schools is in its infancy, a number of successful efforts at both primary and secondary prevention have been documented. Yet, despite these demonstrations, there has not been sufficiently widespread dissemination and implementation. The goals of this chapter are to examine the efforts to prevent mental health problems that have been implemented in our schools, and to delineate those factors that are important for the success of primary prevention programs. This should facilitate future efforts to develop, implement, evaluate, and/or disseminate school programs designed to prevent mental health problems.

This chapter is presented in three major sections: (1) a discussion of resistance to school-based prevention programs; (2) a description of the different types of primary prevention programs that are feasible in schools; and (3) a model for implementing primary prevention in schools. Because the objective is to present both a scholarly and pragmatic view of the topic that will influence practice, case examples will be used to supplement the research literature and to illustrate the points made in the chapter.

RESISTANCE TO PRIMARY PREVENTION

Any professional who has attempted to implement preventive techniques in schools has coped with the frustration of a system that is generally resistant to change and specifically resistant to prevention. Despite a growing body of literature that supports the potential efficacy of prevention, schools cling to a crisis mentality in delivering mental health and other special services. Despite this resistance, preventive techniques must become a priority in our society, and as many have argued previously schools provide an ideal site to promote prevention given their contact with virtually the entire population of young people. Efforts to implement preventive techniques in schools have occurred increasingly in recent years and there has been a concomitant growth in the sophistication and potential effectiveness of these approaches. Yet, it is difficult to convince educators that they need mental health services until a problem is apparent, and it is even more difficult to convince the community to pay for services when they don't see the need. This problem was expressed clearly by a school principal who asked, "How can we fix what ain't broke?" (Lorion, Work, & Hightower, 1984).

Emory Cowen (1977) has argued that resistance to primary prevention has occurred largely because of the diffuseness of the concept. It is difficult to demonstrate the efficacy of a technique the goal of which is to prevent something from occurring. Nevertheless, the concept of prevention has been so appealing historically that it has resulted in numerous premature programmatic efforts. Thus prevention has been implemented before an adequate technology was developed and without adequate research or conceptual models. Prevention programs have been implemented without adequate data on the incidence of the particular maladjustment, without an adequate knowledge base about the disorder including its causes and the factors that maintain it, and without adequate procedures to assess the presence or absence of a particular target behavior. In fact, many prevention programs have been implemented without a clear focus on a target disorder, and generally there has been an emphasis on program development along with an unfortunate deemphasis on evaluation (Lorion, 1983).

One societal factor that inhibits prevention efforts is a widespread preference for the status quo and a general resistance to change of any sort. This is particularly true in institutions like the school because many groups of workers feel that their job security can be threatened by change. This is compounded by the fact that preventive efforts require a shift in the underlying philosophy of our schools. For example, a serious consideration of primary prevention in schools would require changes in such fundamental areas as the curriculum of the school, the structure of schools, and even the underlying purpose of schools as extending beyond the traditional "3Rs."

Primary prevention programs in schools require innovation, and as Seymour Sarason (1971) has pointed out so cogently, innovation is difficult to accomplish in public schools. The politics of schools can lead to miscommunication between innovators and educators when each interprets the innovation as meeting their own needs without thinking clearly about the perspective of the other. Too often this process involves a rush toward acceptance of the proposal without the careful planning that is necessary for success. The result is that even though teachers are frequently the crucial personnel implementing primary prevention techniques, typically they are not consulted seriously during program development. As a result, preventive programs are often imposed on teachers whose natural resistance to change within the educational system is exacerbated by this negative process.

AN EXAMPLE OF INSTITUTIONAL RESISTANCE

The senior author was involved in a prevention project that illustrates this type of resistance, as well as the types of errors that can increase resistance. The broad goal of this project was to help to prevent the development of Special Education problems in schools by getting teachers actively involved in preventive activities. This broad goal was to be accomplished by training teachers to use observation techniques so that they would be able to participate more actively in determining and evaluating the interventions that might be needed to reduce existing problems and prevent the development of more serious problems in the future. For example, after teachers were trained to observe disruptive behavior systematically, they would be more effective in planning and implementing classroom interventions to reduce disruptive behavior.

This project was initiated through the Division of Special Education so that detailed negotiations occurred between that department (particularly its director) and the prevention project. Although sanction for the project was also obtained through the superintendent of schools, this was accomplished verbally through the director of Special Education who implied that there would be no difficulty obtaining support from the superintendent. In retrospect, this was the first mistake. As noted elsewhere (e.g., Meyers, Parsons, & Martin, 1979; Parsons & Meyers, 1984), it is essential that the highest level of administration responsible for a new program be involved during the initial stages of negotiation.

The next step was to initiate a triadic negotiation between the prevention project, the Division of Special Education, and the assistant superintendant in charge of curriculum. This was essential because the project's goal went well beyond special education and involved all regular education teachers. This triadic conference was short but was summarized carefully in writing with the summary being accepted by all parties at the close of the school year. It appeared that the project was set to begin in August. The second mistake was made at this point. No verbal communication occurred to confirm the participants' common understanding of the written summary. As it turned out, each participant had interpreted the document consistent with their own biases and needs. The result was that in the preliminary meeting in August designed to intitiate the project, the assistant superintendant informed the project staff that more than half of the project's time had been allocated to a different districtwide inservice program, which was the new priority of the district.

Earlier direct negotiations with the superintendant might have circumvented this problem. However, this was compounded by the third mistake, which was made at this point. Rather than indicating that the project could not be carried out effectively in this restricted manner, the project staff tried to formulate a compromised version of the program so that it would be accepted for implementation in September. This resulted in an inadequate plan that was doomed to failure. It was negotiated in this manner because the project staff had already invested so much time and energy to work with this school district and because the project staff had its own pressures, independent of the school district, to implement the project as soon as possible.

The fourth error in planning occurred when the project was initiated with the teachers. The first component provided didactic and role-play experiences designed to enhance observation skills that would later be used by teachers in their classrooms. However, because of the compromises made in establishing the project, teachers were not asked for their input regarding training. This proved to be a fatal error resulting in so much teacher resistance that it was impossible to carry out the training satisfactorily. A project's potential for success is affected dramatically by the degree to which those involved with its implementation understand the details of the project and have a sense of ownership for the project.

It was at this late stage that the project staff assessed the errors in planning and decided to revamp the entire program. The one school in the district that had been receptive to the project was selected as a pilot school, and the whole negotiation process was started again. Meetings were set up with the superintendent, assistant superintendent, director of Special Education, and the principal of the proposed pilot school. This group agreed to a plan for intensive negotiation with the faculty of this school to determine the shape of the project. A meeting with the teachers was scheduled, and this meeting was cleared by the teachers' union, which was urged to have formal representation at the meeting (the union had been bypassed in earlier negotiations). The meeting was used to draw out the teachers' feelings about the project to this point and to determine whether agreement could be reached about using the prevention project in this school.

The teachers expressed their desire for skills training that they could use to facilitate their work with particular problem children, and 10 teachers agreed to participate on a trial basis. Even though this was more limited than the broad preventive intents of the program, the staff agreed to this as an entree to the school. Once this aspect of the project was initiated, the program was well received by the participating teachers in the pilot school. All of the teachers who were trained to use observation techniques with specific problem children reported that the observations helped them to plan successful interventions for these children. Once these teachers saw the potential benefits from observing behavior with problem children, they began using these techniques with other children in their class. Five of the teachers did this by choosing one additional child with behavior problems whom they observed. The observations were used to plan interventions that were implemented in all cases and were viewed as successful by 5 of the 6 teachers. The remaining 4 teachers adapted the observation strategies to their entire classrooms and used this as a basis for determining the success of their efforts to improve the behavior of their entire class. As a result, this project influenced all of the participating teachers. All of them were now more likely to use observation strategies as an aid when confronted with a difficult student. Furthermore, 4 of them had already seen the potential preventive impact of this strategy in planning for effective management of the entire class. In this particular example, careful planning and negotiation with the teaching staff required the initial use of secondary and tertiary prevention techniques before the teachers were ready to accept the use of these procedures to accomplish primary prevention goals.

A Summary of Issues Concerning Resistance

A number of general principles concerning resistance to primary prevention must be considered carefully by professionals attempting to implement primary prevention in schools. Many of these have been noted in the prior discussion. This discussion can be summarized by considering techniques to reduce resistance to prevention programs in schools, such as the following 9 principles. These principles are designed to present concrete suggestions for professionals planning to implement prevention programs in schools. Resistance to prevention programs can be minimized when the following is true: (1) there is an adequate knowledge base about the disorder that is to be prevented; (2) there is a clear focus on a target behavior; (3) the innovator understands school culture generally, and the culture of the target school, in particular; (4) the innovator negotiates directly with all relevant administrators, including the highest level of administrator in the organization that is relevant to the project; (5) the innovator takes the necessary time to be sure that all parties understand the proposed project clearly; (6) the prevention staff does not respond to pressures to implement the program in a hurry; (7) the teachers and other staff members are actively involved in determining the prevention project; (8) the prevention project is willing to meet the system's perceived needs first, which often means beginning with secondary and tertiary prevention projects; and (9) the innovator takes active steps to draw out resistance before implementation.

PRIMARY PREVENTION PROGRAMS IN SCHOOLS

Primary prevention as used in this chapter refers to those school programs designed to prevent all children (or an entire subgroup of children) from developing mental health problems. Primary prevention programs are directed toward an entire group of children before there are signs of a developing problem. Thus all children in a school district or potentially vulnerable subgroups would be the focus of these efforts. Examples of vulnerable subgroups include children from single-parent families, or families whose income places them at the poverty level.

There are two basic types of primary prevention programs in schools and it is useful to conceptualize them separately. The first type includes those approaches that seek to promote psychosocial health by developing competence. Strategies designed to increase interpersonal skills, to foster self-esteem, and to develop coping skills are consistent with this type of approach. Success can be assessed directly based on evidence of increased competence related to the intervention. In addition, success can be determined from a reduced incidence of maladjustment.

The second major type of primary prevention strategy is to eliminate the causes or mediators of maladjustment by modifying the environment. These approaches try to use ecological, behavioral, and/or mental health principles as a basis for structuring the environment to reduce stress and to enhance interpersonal relationships. This approach can be assessed based either on evidence that incidence rates have been reduced or on evidence indicating that the environment has been modified.

Building Competence

As indicated earlier, there are two basic approaches to providing primary prevention in schools: building competence and modifying the environment. This section of the chapter will review briefly some of the promising approaches that have been used by schools to prevent maladjustment by building competence. Considered here will be three approaches to building competence. This is not intended as an all-inclusive review of the relevant literature. Instead, a range of approachs has been selected based on two criteria: (1) evidence documenting efficacy of the procedure, and (2) procedures that are viewed as practical to implement. The three approaches to be discussed in this chapter include: (a) teaching interpersonal problem-solving skills, (b) using the school routine to build "strens" (i.e., capacity to cope with stress), and (c) early education programs for children and parents.

TEACHING INTERPERSONAL PROBLEM-SOLVING SKILLS

One approach toward building competence that has received a great deal of attention is the teaching of interpersonal problem-solving skills. This orientation had its basis on Ralph Ojemann's (1969) work developing curricular materials to teach causal thinking to children. Ojemann demonstrated that teaching children to think about behavior in causal terms resulted in strong problem-solving skills and better adjustment. Ojemann developed curricular materials that could be used to teach an entire classroom group about those factors that underly behavior. For example, he was able to teach children to understand the causes of behavior significantly better than controls, and others using his approach with classroom groups have found that these curricular materials can result in greater adjustment and lower anxiety (Alpert, 1983). The basic notion was to use an academic curriculum to teach cognitive skills that could be used by children to contend with social, personal, and interpersonal issues more effectively. The basic questions that need to be asked with this approach include the following:

(1) What are the core skills that provide the basis for social and emotional adjustment?
(2) Can curriculum-related teaching techniques be developed to help children learn these skills?
(3) When a specific skill or competence is taught, will this result in improved adjustment?
(4) When skills or competencies are learned or when emotional adjustment improves, will these changes be maintained?

This approach has been developed in detail by George Spivack and Myrna Shure (1974) at Hahnemann University. Following up Ojemann's work, they teach children skills such as sensitivity to others, awareness of the causal effects of one's behavior on others, the perception of feelings, the development and use of alternative plans, and the awareness of means-end relationships. Means-end relationships refer to the ability to conceptualize the specific sequence of steps necessary to achieve a particular end. The Hahnemann group has worked carefully to develop curricular materials designed to teach these skills to children and they have done substantive research demonstrating the efficacy and potential of this approach. They have demonstrated that two particular cognitive skills consistently relate to behavioral adjustment: the ability to *generate alternative action plans* and the ability to *anticipate consequences* of behavior. They have demonstrated that these problem-solving skills are highest in well-adjusted children, that training with curricular materials can result in increased problem-solving skills, and that improved interpersonal cognitive problem-solving skills are related to improved behavioral adjustment. These findings have occurred consistently for various populations including various handicapping conditions and age groups, and these skills have been found to be independent of intelligence.

A good deal of Shure and Spivack's research has been done with impulsive and inhibited 4-year-old inner-city children who have improved adjustment ratings following training. These children can be trained effectively by both teachers and parents and when parents have been used as trainers an important added effect has been the parents' improved interpersonal problem-solving skills.

The preventive potential of these techniques also has been demonstrated over time. Teacher-trained 4-year-old normal children are less likely than controls to show evidence of problems in kindergarten, and these gains have been maintained for 2 years without further intervention. Moreover, children trained by parents have demonstrated changes in problem-solving skills. It is presumed that this has preventive implications in that changes in the child may be reinforced on an ongoing basis by changes in the mother's parenting style. Moreover, it is likely that there would be a cyclical effect, with changes in the child's behavior also reinforcing changes in the mother's behavior, and as a result it is reasonable to assume that the child's improved problem-solving skills would last years beyond the training program, presumably because of changes in mother-child interaction (Shure & Spivack, 1979).

Many sources summarize research conducted by the Hahneman group, and the reader interested in more detailed information is encouraged to examine the following sources: Shure and Spivack (1978), Spivack, Platt, and Shure (1976) and Spivack and Shure (1974). In addition, specific curricular materials and training manuals can be obtained by practitioners interested in using similar approaches (e.g., Allen, Chinsky, Larcen, & Lochman, & Selinger, 1976; Camp & Bash, 1981; Elardo &

Copper, 1977; Gesten, Apodaca, Rains, Weissberg, & Cowen, 1979; Shure & Spivack, 1974; Spivack & Shure, 1974). In each instance the program is based on a detailed description of the necessary problem-solving steps. One such series of problem-solving steps has been developed by Emory Cowen (Gesten et al., 1979), and we have found these to be useful as a framework to develop materials and procedures for training these skills. The professional beginning to implement this sort of program may do well to start with some of the available pre-packaged curricular materials referred to above. However, once there is sufficient familiarity with the concepts and procedures, some professionals may wish to develop materials specific to their own situation. Although this can require more work, we have found this to be the most effective way to teach social problem-solving skills in the variety of unique school situations we have encountered. Cowen's steps are presented here for those practitioners interested in developing their own materials and programs, and to provide a concrete idea of the types of problem-solving skills that are typically addressed by these programs.

The first skill is to *be aware of upset feelings.* This is Step 1. Problem solving cannot begin until it is recognized that there is a problem to be solved. Children can be taught to be aware of a potential problem once they learn to identify that problem with feelings of anger, sadness, depression, frustration, and so on. Often, children know that they "feel" something, but do not have the ability to identify, label, and disclose these feelings. Consequently, the first part of a training program frequently must teach children to identify their feelings.

Problem definition is the second problem-solving step. Once the child learns to use feelings to identify the general problem area, it is important to define the specific problem in more precise terms. As with any other type of problem, interpersonal problems require precise definition in order to develop useful intervention plans. The third step is to develop a *precise statement of goal(s).* A clear goal is necessary to develop potential solutions; yet many children fail to use this step. In fact, many adults fail to clarify their goal(s) prior to responding to an interpersonal situation.

Steps 4, 5, and 6 are closely related and are crucial to the problem-solving process. Step 4 is labeled *impulse delay* and it requires that the youngster think before acting. Impulsivity is a common problem with children in situations where problem solving was not effective. Although it is difficult for many children to control their impulsivity, this is a skill that can be taught cognitively. Steps 5 and 6 each help to delay impulsivity. Step 5 involves the *generation of alternatives*. As noted earlier, prior research has documented the relationship between this skill and adjustment (e.g., Shure & Spivack, 1978; Spivack & Shure, 1974). When learning this skill children are asked to think of as many solutions as they can in order to solve the problem that they have defined. By generating solutions over time in training sessions, children come to adopt this problem-solving technique in their everyday lives; it becomes a part of their problem-solving repertoire.

Step 6 also helps to delay impulses by requiring the child to *consider the consequences* of his or her behavior. In training children to develop this skill they are asked to think of the different consequences that could possibly occur following each alternative plan. Just like the generation of alternatives, research has demonstrated that the ability to consider the consequences of behavior consistently relates to adjustment.

Step 7 involves *implementation of a plan* to deal with the problem defined in Step 2. During this aspect of training, children are taught to select and implement the best potential plan. Once a plan is initiated it is important that the child learns to evaluate the effects of the plan. Step 8 is to *evaluate the solution*. In those instances when the solution does not work, the child is taught to recycle through the problem-solving process and try again to develop an effective plan of action.

An example of these steps occurred when the second author developed a prevention project designed to reduce the dropout rate in an inner-city high school. This work was initiated because of a crisis involving a 15-year-old girl named Marie who refused to attend school. This was used as a stimulus to discuss with the principal the need for the school to respond in a proactive and preventive manner because school attendance was a problem for large numbers of children in this school. After meetings with the faculty, it was decided that the consultant would colead a group with the chair of the math department designed to help underachieving children. In the past these had been the youngsters who were most frustrating to the school when they dropped out. In initial group meetings the adolescents expressed anger toward parents and the school, noting that there was no value to attending school. Many of the children (and particularly Marie) noted their boredom in school, and Marie brought the discussion to a head when she exclaimed angrily that there "was nothing wrong with me...except that everybody is bugging me."

Although these youngsters were generally quick to identify their anger toward the school, they did not recognize that their "boredom" might actually reflect mild depression. Step 1 was implemented by teaching the group to identify their feelings. As a result, they became aware that many of their feelings about school were tied to self-doubt and a sense of hopelessness in school rather than to boredom or anger. In addition, Marie acknowledged that she felt as if she was constantly disappointing her parents, and this exacerbated her sense of hopelessness.

After clarifying their feelings the second step, problem definition, was initiated. A general problem was accepted by the group in that all of the students felt that they underachieved in school and wanted to do better. As a part of this process of problem definition the group was encouraged to identify those factors that supported their underachievement. Some of these factors included their self-doubt, their poor study skills, and their habit of cutting school. The third step is to determine a precise goal. The most generally stated goal was to attend college following high school, and some even indicated a long-term wish to earn various scholastic honors. A specific goal was accepted by the entire group: to earn at least a B on their next exam.

In an effort to achieve this specific goal, steps 4, 5 and 6 were implemented with regard to "cutting school." Step 4, impulse delay, requires that the youngster think before acting. The group was taught to delay the impulse to cut class or to avoid a home-work assignment. Each time they had one of these impulses they were instructed to say to themselves, "I should stop and think before doing anything that might interfere with my school goals. I can do this if I wait at least 5 minutes and if I begin to consider consequences and alternatives." At this point Steps 5 and 6 were implemented in an effort to teach the children to consider alterna-tive plans of behavior and to consider the consequences of each plan. This was done by having the group imagine those instances when they considered cutting school. First they were asked to brainstorm the possible consequences that resulted when they cut school (e.g., they missed key work necessary to understand the next test, their teachers developed a negative attitude toward them, other students became less likely to offer help, they dis-appointed their parents, and they lost privileges at home). Next, the group was asked to consider alternative plans. This proved to be difficult because the only alternative they could generate at first was, "Go to school." This alternative was limited because it was not perceived as rewarding. As a result the group was taught to generate more detailed alternatives such as, "Go to school in the morning, go to lunch at a local restaurant with friends, go to the Recreation Center after school, and study with a friend after dinner." After the group became more effective at developing useful alternatives, they were taught to consider the consequences of these plans by brainstorming as a group. In this way they were taught to determine the potential efficacy of each plan.

Steps 7 and 8 involve the implementation of a plan and its evaluation. Initially this was taught through role play techniques, having each youngster take at least one turn role playing the plan that they thought had the most potential to be effective and then evaluating its efficacy. This was done by using other group members to play key parts such as a parent, a teacher, or a friend. After the role plays each youngster was given feed-back and there was a discussion of the strengths and weaknesses of their implementation of the plan as well as the evaluation. Then each group member was given a homework assignment to try out the technique the next time they had an impulse to cut school. These real efforts were then discussed to further consolidate the problem-solving steps that had been learned.

The last step in training was to teach the group that these problem-solving steps could be used to resolve a variety of life problems. This was done through discussion and through the active use of these same steps to help solve a variety of other problems generated by group members during the year. It is important to note that the grades and attendance of all but one of the group members improved dramatically during the year. In particular, Marie's behavior improved with no further mention of her desire to drop out of school, and, because she had been the stimulus for the project, this helped to demonstrate to the rest of the school the potential of problem solving as an effective approach to prevention.

USING THE SCHOOL ROUTINE TO BUILD "STRENS"

About twenty years ago William Hollister coined the term "strens" in a discussion of primary prevention. His basic notion was that successful exposure to minor stressful experiences would build the individual's capacity to cope with stress in the future. He suggested that this capacity to cope with future stress could be labeled "strens," a term that signifies the individual's strength in dealing with stress. This is a concept with pragmatic implications for prevention in schools because it results in ideas that can be implemented inexpensively.

We have found that three particular issues have pragmatic implications for the development of strens in school children. These three issues include learning to deal with loss, learning to deal with conflict, and exposure to developmental crises. They each have substantial preventive implications for schools because the school experience is filled with repeated exposure to each type of stress.

Loss is experienced by the school-aged child in many different ways: for example, loss of parental support and comfort begins when the child is required to attend school for the first time; loss of friends in school as they move on to other schools and locations; the death of a classroom pet or mascot; and the sense of loss experienced when making the transition from one teacher to another following grade promotion. Each of these types of loss can be a source of stress for the school-aged child. Although these "losses" are generally less than devastating, they do increase stress and provide school personnel with an opportunity to "teach" the child more adequate coping skills. As the child builds strens in this way he or she can become more competent and adaptive in later life when confronted with intensive stressors such as separation, divorce, or death.

An example of this approach occurred in a nursery school class where a gerbil was found dead by the student teacher. The student teacher was concerned about children, whom she thought would be upset if they found out. Her solution was to replace the gerbil secretly before school the next day. Fortunately, the teacher saw this as an opportunity for the children to learn about death and to develop some skills in coping with loss. Despite the student teacher's objections, an encounter was engineered in which the children discovered the dead animal. They examined the body, discussed the meaning of death, and tested their assumptions about death. Some discovered that the gerbil did not move, others indicated that it was not as warm as it had been previously, and still others found that it did not respond in any way to prodding. They discussed the fact that being dead meant that this animal would not come back to life, and some of them expressed their sadness. Not only did they learn a "lesson" with important cognitive components, they also may have begun to develop their capacity to cope with loss as they learned more about their feelings in this situation.

The teacher in the preceding example implemented a primary prevention technique as a routine part of her interaction with students when an opportunity arose. She did not have a huge grant to support a complicated primary prevention project and she was not part of a large staff whose major function was to provide primary prevention services. Yet this type of intervention has the potential to be highly effective because it can be an ongoing part of the day-to-day educational program. In fact, educators may be the most crucial factor in the successful implementation of primary prevention in schools. This is an important factor to acknowledge because it implies that educators rather than mental health professionals are often responsible for the success of primary prevention in schools.

Conflict is an ongoing part of the school experience. There is conflict between students and students, students and teachers, students and their parents, and so on. Students must learn to deal with these different sources of conflict so that they can function most effectively in school as well as in later life. If teachers see these situations as learning opportunities for their students, they can create an atmosphere in which the school is a laboratory setting where a student can learn and practice positive skills for coping effectively with conflict. The types of conflict experienced in school vary from physical confrontation between students, to verbal confrontation between students, or between teachers and students. Each of these can be used to help children learn and develop coping skills.

Interpersonal conflict generally involves a struggle between a least two parties who have incompatible goals. Schools can help children deal with conflict by teaching them to move from a "win-lose" orientation to a "no-lose" strategy. In a win-lose situation it is inevitable that one party must lose. To implement a "no-lose" strategy it is necessary to find a solution in which everyone's needs are met.

An example occurred in an inner-city elementary school when 2 fifth graders were fighting over who was going to clean the erasers for the teacher. The educator's first impulse might be to say something like, "Because you are fighting you can both sit down and Barbara will get to do the job." This is clearly a "lose-lose" strategy. Instead, this situation provides an opportunity to teach the children how to use a "no-lose" strategy. Following this model the teacher asked, "What is the problem?" The children shouted simultaneously, "It is my turn to clean the erasers." The teacher asked each child, "What happened?" After getting a separate answer from each youngster the teacher pointed out how they set up a situation in which they would both lose. Then she asked, "What else could you have done?

How could you have worked this out to satisfy both of you?'' After brainstorming for a few minutes the youngsters realized that they could have shared the job this time. The teacher then used this as an opportunity to instruct the entire class in ''no-lose'' strategies for dealing with conflict situations.

By repeatedly using examples such as this one to instruct the entire class in the difference between ''win-lose'' and ''no-lose'' strategies, a simple approach to implementing a preventive program designed to promote positive strategies for dealing with conflict was implemented. This can be done by teaching the class the following framework for dealing with conflict. Whenever it is possible to have a class discussion following a conflict situation, this framework serves as a basis for the discussion. The 6-step framework for conflict resolution includes the following: (1) define what each person wants or needs, (2) use brainstorming to generate possible solutions, (3) evaluate the solutions in terms of practicality and effectiveness, (4) try the solution, (5) evaluate effectiveness of the solution, and (6) praise yourself and the other person for good conflict resolution. In addition to discussing these steps with the class after conflict situations occur in school, role play techniques are used to try out ''no-lose'' strategies in potentially difficult situations, and students are given homework assignments to try out these strategies outside of school.

Developmental crises present another opportunity to promote the acquisition of strens by school children. We have found four developmental crises to be particularly useful in this context. *School entrance* is the first crisis that is confronted by all school children and it has multiple implications for primary prevention. As noted earlier, it is a significant opportunity for the child to learn to cope with separation from parents. It is also an opportunity for children to learn to cope with change in routine because it represents such a dramatic change in schedule for the child. Finally, when children first enter school they often have one of their first experiences with competition and the pressure to achieve. This presents an excellent early opportunity for the nursery school or kindergarten teacher to teach the child strategies to cope more effectively with pressures for achievement.

A second related crisis is *school achievement pressure* in later elementary school. Frequently the transition to increased work demands occurs in fourth grade as the demands for independent work and the sheer amounts of homework and class work are increased dramatically. This is a point where achievement anxiety can become a serious problem and students need to learn skills to cope with these pressures. Cognitive procedures can be taught to children so that they learn to evaluate their performance demands more objectively. Also, students need to learn and develop organizational skills so they have the capacity to cope more effectively with the demands for independent work.

The third significant developmental crisis that we have found to be useful for prevention is the *transition from elementary school to junior high school.* Not only is there a move from the security of elementary school to the larger junior high—with lots of new students, new academic demands, and a new educational structure—but this is also that awkward age at which students emerge into adolescence. Students need to develop skills to cope with the new demands of these situations, and they need to learn to cope with the physical changes that are occurring. Moreover, this is a period that emphasizes peer relations and it is an important time to learn productive strategies for coping with a variety of new interpersonal demands occurring at this stage. An example of an approach designed to promote strens for junior high students is presented later in this chapter in the section on Reducing Stress.

The last developmental stage that we have used to develop preventive programs is the *transition toward independence,* which occurs in high school. As high school students become more independent they confront situations that they often must solve on their own. Most notably, these include new exposure to drugs, alcohol, and sex. It is an age when values become particularly important, and they need to develop the capacity to understand and assess their own values while not being shaken from them by pressure from peers. School experiences such as classroom group discussions about values, teacher reactions to incidents involving students, and student-teacher relationships can all be used to promote productive development of independent decision-making skills by high school students. It is also possible to establish preventive counseling groups to deal with these issues; however, it is important to remember that effective classroom teachers can deal with these issues on an ongoing basis throughout the school day and throughout the year.

Each of these developmental crises as well as the general issues of loss and conflict have unique potential in facilitating the development of coping capacity by building strens, and they can each be used by classroom teachers as a basis for developing classroom strategies for accomplishing these goals. By developing strategies that can be implemented routinely as a part of classroom instruction there is a dramatic potential to produce a generation of students with greater capacity to cope with stress. However, frequently educators do not see this as an appropriate goal and often they do not see these as crucial educational opportunities. As a result, many opportunities for teaching coping skills are probably lost in the schools. It is essential that educational philosophy is broadened so that the development of social/emotional competence becomes one of its key goals.

It has been noted throughout this section that teachers are the key personnel necessary for a school to use developmental crises in a systematic way to promote social/emotional development and to prevent mental health problems in the future. Because of their regular contact with children, teachers are often in an excellent position to use the various crises (school entrance, academic pressure in middle elementary school, entrance to junior high school, adolescence) to facilitate growth. In order to do this systematically, it is important that the school provide in-service training so that teachers become aware of these crises and their potential value as an opportunity to teach coping skills to children. In-service training can also be used to provide the skills needed to implement some of the specific programs mentioned above. Once in-service has been provided, the school must provide consultative support to help teachers implement these types of activities. This can be provided through the school psychologist, the school counselor, the school principal, a senior teacher experienced in these approaches, or a support group composed of teachers who meet regularly to discuss their efforts in these areas.

EARLY EDUCATION PROGRAMS

Much work has been done demonstrating the potential efficacy of a variety of early education programs designed to provide stimulation and enrichment as well as added learning. These programs have been offered to groups of people in danger of educational failure—most frequently to economically disadvantaged groups. Many early interventions programs have documented striking improvement in academic, social, and emotional indicators, and some studies have documented increased IQ scores. The first massive effort in this connection was the federally funded Operation Head Start, which experimented with several different models of curriculum to provide early childhood education (e.g., behavioral models, cognitive/developmental models, personal growth models). A general conclusion from the evaluations of Head Start suggests that each of these broad approaches to early intervention demonstrated gains that varied depending on the program's emphasis. For example, whereas behavioral and cognitive models tended to report cognitive or achievement gains, personal growth models reported gains in social/emotional areas.

Another important finding is that these gains were short term, but that they could be maintained by providing similar follow-up programs in elementary school. This hypothesis was confirmed with Project Follow Through, which was a successful federally funded program designed to continue in early elementary school the programs that had been offered by Head Start. One conclusion reached from the evaluations of Operation Head Start and Project Follow Through is that parent involvement is a key factor to ensure success of early education programs.

Various early childhood education programs have been implemented subsequent to these earlier efforts, usually beginning at about 2 or 3 years of age and continuing at least through kindergarten. It has been found that there is a substantial potential for preventive effects (Lazar, Darlington, & Associates, 1982;

Pierson, Walker, & Tivnan, 1984; Weber, Foster, & Weikart, 1978; Weikart, 1984). For example, they found that there are fewer retentions, fewer children placed in special education, and fewer school dropouts as a result of these programs. Cost-benefit analyses suggest reduced costs of special education, fewer school dropouts higher earnings for graduates, and fewer court convictions (e.g., Weber et al., 1978). One longitudinal analysis conducted by Weikart (1984) even found a lower birthrate for those who had been pupils in the cognitive model preschool program, resulting in Weikart's facetious claim that preschool intervention may even be a promising form of birth control.

To summarize, early education programs can have long-term results that have important preventive implications. To obtain these results it is necessary to involve parents actively so that there is support in the home, and it is necessary to continue providing the same type of educational services, including screening and referral services for children with potential learning problems. The particular curricular approach can vary depending upon the goals and philosophy of the program (i.e., behavioral, cognitive, or personal growth models), because there is evidence that each of these models can be effective in achieving certain goals. It may also be important to provide training for teachers to increase their skills, and to provide an improved teacher pupil ratio by using teacher aides. This would allow for more individualized attention to children under any of the different models of curriculum. Although this can require special financial and administrative support to be implemented effectively, it is possible to implement some aspects of the program at minimal costs using parent volunteers and other volunteers from the community (e.g., senior citizens). Moreover, cost-benefit analyses justify these costs given the potent preventive effects that have been demonstrated. It is beyond the scope of this chapter to provide a detailed description of the strategies needed to implement an effective early childhood program geared toward the above preventive results. However, the practitioner interested in these details including information about the curriculum, the procedures for training staff, and other specific strategies necessary for implementation is referred to the following sources: Hauser-Cram and Pierson (1981), Hohmann, Banet, and Weikart (1979), Stone, Pendleton, and Vaill (1980), and Yurchak (1975).

Modifying the Environment

Until recently the mental health fields have generally ignored the potential of social systems. However, there is a growing body of evidence indicating that social environments can have a profound impact on mental health (e.g., Moos, 1973, 1974b, 1979). There are two basic approaches to modify the environment: (1) promote a positive social climate in either the school or the classroom, and (2) reduce stress. These two approaches are described briefly in the two following sections.

(1) Improving Climate: Barker and Gump (1964) were among the first to study systematically the effects of school environment, and at this point a large body of evidence suggests a variety of social, emotional, and academic effects associated with different components of school climate. It has been found that factors associated with classroom climate affect student satisfaction, personal development, and achievement. In addition, a variety of schoolwide factors can affect behavior and grades. Physical characteristics of the school, cultural values, and school morale can all have an impact both on grades and on the behavior of students, and some researchers (e.g., Barker and Gump, 1964) have found greater incidence of behavior problems in large schools. They may occur because students in small schools are more likely to participate, to take responsibility for decisions, and to have their personal needs met. Some additional school characteristics that may be important include shared activities between teachers and students and productive teacher-administration relationships.

Moos and his associates at Stanford have developed a series of scales designed to assess various social environments including school and classroom, and they have begun to investigate the impact of environmental climate on attitudes, behavior adaptation, health, and mental health. Three factors have emerged consistently that describe social climates in a stable manner: (1) relational, (2) goal oriented, and (3) system maintenance and change factors.

Relational factors in schools include involvement, affiliation, and support. Involvement refers to student attentiveness in class, their participation in class discussion, and their interest in class activities. Affiliation indicates the degree of student friendship expressed in school, and this includes how students enjoy working together and the degree to which they help each other. Support refers particularly to the interest, trust, and friendship teachers show toward students, as well as the degree to which they are willing to help students. In general these factors facilitate the personal development of students.

Goal-oriented factors in schools include task orientation and competition. Task orientation refers to the importance given to task completion and the degree to which teachers stick to the subject matter. Competition implies an emphasis on grades where it is recognized that good grades are difficult to obtain. Achieving good grades occurs through direct competition with others according to this dimension.

System maintenance and change factors include order and organization, rule clarity, teacher control, and innovation. Order and organization involves an emphasis on orderly behavior as well as the organization of assignments and class activities. Rule clarity stresses clear rules where students understand precisely the consequences of not following rules. Teacher control refers to the degree to which rules are enforced and the severity of consequences for breaking rules. Innovation involves the variety of activities planned by teachers as well as those activities that are unusual. It also refers to the degree to which students contribute to planning class activities.

Moos's initial research has revealed six types of secondary school classes. These include *innovation-oriented* classes that emphasize innovation, teacher-student interaction, student-student interaction, and variety and change. These classes have little task orientation as well as unclear rules and procedures. The second type of class is labeled *structured relationship oriented*. These classes emphasize student interaction and participation, and student involvement. However, they also emphasize clarity of rules and procedures, and organized activities. The third type of classes are *supportive task oriented*. These classes emphasize academic objectives and teacher support, but provide for little student interaction during class or participation in planning. The fourth type of class is *supportive competition oriented,* and this type focuses on competition in a friendly context, high organization and rule clarity, with a deemphasis on teacher control. The fifth type is referred to as *unstructured competition oriented.* This type emphasizes task orientation and competition, but deemphasizes all the other components of class climate. The sixth, and final, type of class revealed in this research is labeled *control oriented.* This type emphasizes teacher control to the exclusion of all the other dimensions of class climate.

A review of this research reveals four major findings: (1) Relationship- and innovation-oriented classes promote the social and personal growth of students, while developing student interest in the subject matter and satisfaction with school. However, these dimensions are not sufficient to facilitate achievement. (2) High achievement gains are likely in classes that emphasize goal-oriented dimensions (i.e., task orientation and competition) and maintenance dimensions (organization and clarity of rules). However, when these classes are low in warmth they do not facilitate student morale or creativity. (3) Control-oriented classes that deemphasize the other dimensions do not facilitate personal or social growth and do not result in achievement gains. Instead, they are frequently associated with alienation and dissatisfaction on the part of students. (4) Finally, gains on measures of achievement are related to classroom climate based on a combination of dimensions. Gains are likely when there are supportive, warm relationships, with an emphasis on academic goals and tasks, and with a clear, orderly, and well-structured classroom environment. This combination of dimensions also can promote creativity and social/personal growth.

The implications for prevention are straightforward. Schools can promote positive adjustment and reduce mental health problems by establishing environments based on the above factors. The greatest potential for prevention occurs with schools that emphasize each of the three major dimensions (i.e., relationship oriented, goal oriented, and systems maintenance). As is the case so frequently, these preventive activities require knowledge, understanding, and cooperation on the part of teachers and school administrators. Without their support and cooperation, these prevention efforts cannot be successful.

An example of this approach was used by Parsons when consulting to a secondary school with students who had negative attitudes toward school. One math teacher had particularly serious problems including frequent fighting, damaged school property, inattentiveness and disruption in the classroom, and a general resistance to educational tasks. The agreement to provide help to this teacher was followed first by informal observations in his classes. This was followed by a detailed interview with the teacher who agreed to administer Moos's (1974a) Classroom Environment Scale to all students in his classes. The data suggested clearly that his classrooms could be characterized as "control oriented." The teacher was perceived as authoritarian, the students did not feel actively involved in class activities, they felt like they had no input into what went on in the classroom, and they did not feel support from either the teacher or other students in this competitive atmosphere.

This information was presented to the teacher who then spent several sessions working with the consultant to plan ways in which he could increase the goal-oriented focus, increase the support provided to students in the class, and increase student involvement in class activities. The result was that the incidence of classroom disruption decreased whereas student time on tasks increased, and this was generally true of all but one class (the remedial math group composed of the most difficult students in the school). Follow-up during the following year revealed that this teacher's increased competence was maintained over time, and he was even able to use these goal-oriented and relationship oriented techniques to work more effectively with his new remedial group.

(2) Reducing Stress. The environment can be modified to reduce stress. Earlier we described techniques tht increase the child's ability to cope with stress by building "strens." In contrast, this approach seeks to modify the environment to reduce or eliminate unnecessary stress. For example, when a youngster has a memory deficit, teaching strategies that build in memory supports to facilitate the child's learning can reduce stress. Stress can also be reduced in social situations by using teaching strategies based on cooperative principles that encourage children to work together by teaching the skills needed for productive cooperation and by structuring group projects that facilitate cooperative efforts (Johnson & Johnson, 1980). Perhaps one of the most useful approaches to reducing stress by altering the environment is to develop networks designed to provide support for students. This is implemented in schools in various ways. One approach is to establish after school activities in which students from different classes and grades work together on an area of joint interest (e.g., the student newspaper). This is one way that students can find out about each other's strengths and use them to get support from each other.

Formal cross-age networks can be particularly helpful for both old and young children. For example, Bower (1964) has presented the idea of using children at one developmental level (e.g., junior high school students) to work as tutors with young children in elementary school, and we have found this to be particularly useful because of its multiple effects. This helps young children to benefit from the experience of older children and to learn that older children are willing to help. It also provides support that the young child can sometimes call on outside of the formal tutoring relationship. At the same time, the emerging adolescent who faces his or her own social/personal problems at this age can be helped to deal more effectively with these problems simply through the process of helping another child.

An important consideration to ensure the efficacy of this program is in choosing the tutors. Although any junior high aged youngster might be able to profit from the program, it is important to select volunteers whose schedules will permit a regular commitment to the tutoring process along with one day per week after school for training. It is also advisable to avoid using those individuals who display emotional problems unless staff are available to monitor their work closely. This program includes careful training of the tutors on a weekly basis. The training can be conducted by anyone on the staff who has the time and expertise. Because these meetings occur after school, it would be possible for a teacher to lead the group; however, frequently this role is taken by the school counselor. Initially they meet in a small group to learn about child development and child management strategies. This provides the background that is necessary for them to work effectively with the behavior problems of the young children they will tutor.

Once the tutees are selected, each tutor receives individual instruction regarding the area in which they will provide tutoring (e.g., math). During this portion of training the tutors are taught the key concepts they will teach, they are provided with specific lessons they will use, which include concrete material developed by the teacher, and they are encouraged to develop one "lesson" on their own, including the preparation of the necessary material. Once tutoring begins the tutors are "supervised" in a small group of about 5 tutors. During this time they report on their work, focusing particularly on any problems they encounter. By learning about child development and by sharing their varied tutorial experiences in a small group, they can make substantial personal gains, particularly when they discuss the difficult behaviors displayed by the tutees. At the same time this establishes a support group of junior high school students that extends beyond immediate friendship networks.

The above procedures represent just one example of an effective approach to modifying the school environment to reduce the stress associated with school transitions. Another example has been designed to facilitate the transition to high school. This program is designed (1) to reduce the stress associated with the high degree of change and complexity of this new environment; and (2) to increase the social support provided by peers and teachers. Research investigating the efficacy of this program reflected preventive effects that were statistically significant (Felner, Ginter, & Primavera, 1982).

Specifically, this program included two major elements. First, there was a systematic effort to restructure the role of the homeroom teacher so that these teachers, who had daily contact with the students, serve many of the functions traditionally associated with school guidance counselors. For example, these teachers advised the students in selecting classes, contacted the family following student absences, and counseled the students regarding personal difficulties. This increased the emotional support from the teaching staff, it increased students' feelings of accountability, and it increased student accessibility to information about school rules and expectations.

The second major element of the program was to reorganize the social system by assigning students to academic classes from the same small pool of students in the school. This introduced considerably greater stability to the peer group; this was designed to increase the support provided from peers while reducing the constant change traditionally associated with this new social environment.

This section of the chapter has presented two examples of modifying the school environment that reduced stress associated with school transitions by increasing social support and using the concept of networks. A common feature of these approaches is that they are intuitively appealing as practical approaches that can be implemented realistically within the context of schools and that do not require a dramatic increase in financial resources. Moreover, these are just examples of many similar ideas that can be developed by practitioners in response to the unique circumstances in each professional situation.

A MODEL FOR DEVELOPING
PRIMARY PREVENTION PROGRAMS IN SCHOOLS

Emory Cowen (1984) has developed a structural model for program development focused on primary prevention. This model can be applied to schools in order to ensure that primary prevention programs have a maximum probability of success. The model conceptualizes five distinct steps that must be followed for successful program development.

(1) Identify the Program's Generative Base

Too often primary prevention programs are implemented in schools because they are the latest fad or for political reasons. Frequently these programs sound good but are not based on a solid conceptual foundation. As a result, there is often failure in program implementation simply due to inadequate conceptualization. As Cowen (1984) has argued, "If the generative step is omitted there is the danger of developing (and perhaps conducting very well) interventions that are doomed before they ever start—in other words, of doing the wrong things perfectly well."

The generative base for a program is dependent upon knowledge. For primary prevention in schools two types of knowledge have been conceptualized and discussed previously: (1) knowledge about the relationship among certain skills, areas of competence or experience, and adjustment; and (2) knowledge about the relationship between various environmental factors and stress, and their impact on adjustment. As data accumulate documenting that certain competencies relate to adjustment, or that certain environmental factors relate to adjustment, effective plans for primary prevention programs can be developed. For example, earlier in this chapter literature was reviewed suggesting a relationship between classroom climate and adjustment of the learner (e.g., Moos, 1979); another set of studies was reviewed documenting a relationship between interpersonal-cognitive problem-solving skills and adjustment in children (i.e., Shure & Spivack, 1978, 1979). This provides a knowledge base that helps to generate ideas about primary prevention programs to modify classroom climate and to improve social problem-solving skills.

(2) Translate Knowledge Base into Guiding Program Concepts

Once data have established relationships to adjustment, a concept can be formed regarding a prevention program that will have some chance to succeed. For example, after deciding to establish a program to improve classroom climate, it is necessary to decide which of the three major areas of climate to address (e.g., relational factors, goal-oriented factors, and system maintenance and change factors). Because existing research suggests that a balanced focus on all three areas has a maximum opportunity to facilitate both learning and adjustment, the guiding concept would be to focus the prevention program on all three areas.

(3) Developing a Workable Program Technology

Once the general concept of a program has been developed, it becomes necessary to spell out the step-by-step details of the program. In determining the specific procedures five points are particularly important.

(1) Maintain a clear awareness of the characteristics of the target population, with a particular emphasis on developmental levels and readiness for change. As indicated earlier, this would include knowledge about the incidence of the target problem in this population to help guage the need for intervention as well as its effectiveness.

(2) Develop a thorough understanding of the school's characteristics as these may affect the intervention plans. This would include an analysis of the characteristics of the particular school in which the intervention will take place as well as the entire school district. Seymour Sarason (1971) has documented how the unique characteristics of each school as well as its fundamental attitudes concerning mental health can have significant effects on the school's acceptance of innovations—particularly innovations associated with the prevention of mental health problems. Additional school characteristics that require attention include the size of the school and the types of funding available. Generally, when it is possible to help the school obtain external funds to support a new program, the chances of acceptance are much greater; when the district will have to use its own funds acceptance is more difficult. This often presents a serious problem in schools because good innovative programs are dif-

ficult to implement on a long-term basis with temporary external funding sources. Therefore, when helping to negotiate for external funding, it is important to suggest that the school gradually provide increasing funds to support the program over time so that when external funds run out the program can be maintained based on support from the school district.

As pointed out in the example earlier in this chapter, it is essential to understand the power structure of the school clearly, to negotiate with the highest level of the administration from the onset, to include all relevant administrators, and to include teachers and representatives from the teacher's union early in the negotiations for a prevention project. The larger the school district, the more likely it is that miscommunication may occur. It is crucial that care be taken to communicate both verbally and in writing, and to check frequently to be certain that all parties have the same understanding about the project.

(3) In order to develop a workable program it is also important to consider carefully who is initiating the idea because this can have a significant impact on any efforts to implement prevention programs in schools. An external consultant may have to use the most formal means of communication. On the other hand, an internal consultant may have more informal communication networks established throughout the district that may facilitate the project. The extreme example of this is the classroom teacher who wishes to implement a prevention program on his or her own. As long as the program does not violate a school norm and does not upset parents, this can usually be accomplished fairly easily. In contrast, the external consultant would need to communicate formally with the superintendant (and possibly the school board), other relevant administrators from central office, the school principal, the district's teacher's union, the teacher's in the target school, the parents, and so on.

One way to conceptualize the difference between the internal and external consultant in this context is in terms of "expert power" and "referent power" (Meyers et al., 1979). *Expert power* is the ability to influence another person based on the degree to which he or she perceives you as possessing the expertise needed to solve the problem. *Referent power* is the ability to influence another person based on the degree to which he or she identifies with you. Generally, the external consultant will begin with greater expert power and may need to develop referent power, thus emphasizing the need to communicate throughout all levels of the district. On the other hand, the internal consultant is likely to begin with greater referent power and may need to emphasize the development of expert power by demonstrating the efficacy of the program.

(4) One factor that can have dramatic effects on the success of a primary prevention program in schools concerns the variety of personnel who may have to work with the program, and the problem of "professional turf." For example, if school counselors wish to run social problem-solving groups with children, there will be minimal problems implementing the program once it is accepted by the principal, the teachers, and the parents. In this instance there is minimal reliance on other school personnel to carry out the program. On the other hand, a school program designed to provide social skills groups *run by a teacher* in each classroom in the school requires cooperation from all of the classroom teachers. Moreover, if this schoolwide social skills program were proposed by some group other than the school counselors (e.g., the school psychologist, classroom teachers, an external consultant), it could be a complicated political task to obtain acceptance of the project. A social skills program might be thought of as a form of group counseling, and as a result of feelings regarding professional turf, the counselors could easily block this well-intended project. Similar concerns about turf can arise between regular and special education. As illustrated by the example presented in the earlier section on resistance, it is important to be clear about the involvement and commitments made by each group. One of the most important skills for ensuring the success of prevention programs is the ability to facilitate effective communication between the relevant groups of school professionals.

(5) The last point relevant to developing a workable program is to consider the emphasis of school administrators on

a balanced budget. There is great reluctance to spend money on projects that appear to be frills with no concrete educational gains and no clear advantages in terms of cost-benefit analyses. As a result, it is important to have a sound grasp of the research base for the program. But, in addition, it is essential to provide information about the cost effectiveness of the program. It would be useful to have information available about the efficacy of such programs at reducing future costs of special education, reducing the numbers of future arrests, reducing future costs for community mental health centers and psychiatric hospitals, and so on.

(4) Conducting the Program

Once the program has been conceived and carefully planned, it must be carried out. The effectiveness of this process will depend upon careful attention to mechanisms designed to keep those responsible for the program in constant touch with the program. This requires a continual monitoring of the program to assess its strengths and weaknesses so that necessary changes can be made. To do this it will be important to build in mechanisms to help identify problems. For example, during training there should be regular meetings to ensure that training is proceeding smoothly. Similarly, staff meetings should be held regularly during implementation to review the program. There should be regular observations of the program to be sure that it is working as planned. There should be periodic process reports from the project staff to pick up on any problems, and consultation should be available routinely to those on the staff responsible for implementation. Thus, for example, if teachers are required to implement social skills groups in their classrooms, it is crucial to provide adequate training, monitor the groups through periodic observations, obtain process reports from the teachers in a way that does not overburden their already busy schedule, and provide regular consultation support to brainstorm alternative approaches to those problems that occur. Because these steps all require time, it will be essential that this part of the project be negotiated thoroughly with all relevant parties prior to implementation.

(5) Evaluating the Program

In order to ensure the long-term success of a prevention program, it is essential that program evaluation data are gathered. This will help to demonstrate efficacy of the program that will be necessary to obtain continued support. Moreover, for the evaluation to be effective, it must be planned from the outset. Too often, well-designed programs are planned and initiated without adequate program evaluation built in. Then as the program nears completion and there is a desire to seek additional support, a last-minute effort is made to evaluate the program. This approach to evaluation is generally filled with so many problems that the eventual findings are of limited value and may jeopardize continued funding for an otherwise good program.

In order to plan an adequate evaluation it is important to be sure that measures for the target variables are available that have adequate reliability and validity and can be administered within the practical constraints of the school program. It is also necessary to be certain that the available measures are appropriate to the population of concern (e.g., measures for high school students might not be appropriate for use with a preschool population and vice versa). One of the most frequent evaluation errors is to use measures that do not assess the variables that the program is designed to modify. Under these circumstances the evaluation methodology may look sophisticated, but it is doomed to failure because the measure used would be unlikely to be responsive to the intervention.

Finally, it is important to have multiple data sources and to assess the program's efficacy based on a convergence of these different data. This should include longitudinal studies to determine whether initial findings are maintained over time because long-term effects are one of the most important aspects of prevention programs.

SUMMARY AND CONCLUSIONS

This chapter has pointed out that a substantial research base exists indicating the potential efficacy of primary prevention programs in schools. A range of primary prevention programs that have been implemented successfully in schools was reviewed, and it was stressed that classroom teachers often can implement small-scale prevention programs on an informal basis. It was noted that despite the mounting data base, there is still considerable resistance to primary prevention in the schools. Although numerous reasons for this problem were discussed, a model for implementing primary prevention was presented that may help to reduce this resistance.

There are several ideas that may be particularly useful to the school practitioner trying to overcome resistance to primary prevention in schools. These are discussed here by way of conclusion. Some of these points are made here for the first time, but most of them derive from the material presented earlier in this chapter.

(1) It may be necessary to implement secondary prevention programs before gaining acceptance for primary prevention programs. In some schools secondary prevention efforts may be more acceptable than primary prevention, resulting in less resistance. It is beyond the scope of this chapter to review the literature on secondary prevention in schools; the interested reader may consult some of the following sources: Cowen (1977, 1980), Hagin (1980), Lorion et al. (1984), Meyers et al. (1979), and Parsons and Meyers (1984).

(2) It may sometimes be necessary to develop alternative units within the school system to provide the services that others refuse to deliver. Irwin Hyman (1971) has referred to this as developing parallel systems, and one example might be to hire a temporary team of people to implement social skills groups in a school. Once the pragmatic efficacy of this program can be demonstrated, it might be more likely that others from within the system will use the program.

A related idea is to find internal personnel who can be trained as trainers (referred to by Hyman as "turn-keys"). These turn-keys would then train others in the system to implement the program. By using this concept the school is more likely to take ownership of the project and implement it on a long-term basis. At the same time, this approach can be practical because it does not require immediate acceptance and implementation by large numbers of personnel within the system.

(3) Of course, some programs may be implemented most efficiently by people outside of the system. In these instances the program may be most successful by hiring other mental health professionals or by hiring nonprofessional personnel who will be trained to carry out the program. This latter orientation has been used with great success by Cowen (1980).

(4) As noted throughout different sections of this chapter, it is essential that negotiations are conducted clearly with all relevant personnel. Implicit in this process of negotiation is the notion that those responsible for program implementation will be willing and voluntary participants in the program. Our experience has been that prevention programs imposed on unwilling school personnel have been doomed to failure.

(5) Finally, as implied in the previous section of this chapter, program evaluation is essential to successful implementation of primary prevention programs. It helps to demonstrate program effectiveness to administrators, parents, and funding sources, and, equally important, it can be used to help the staff learn from past mistakes. Various program evaluation techniques help to provide data that can be used to make programmatic decisions to improve future efforts.

Schools provide the ideal setting to implement primary prevention techniques. However, ill-conceived programs without carefully designed evaluation plans will have negative long-term effects in that they may reduce support for these programs and increase resistance. Therefore, this chapter has attempted to make the case that if the practitioner wishes to implement primary prevention programs in schools, he or she must proceed with careful attention to the principles outlined in this chapter. The technology is available to implement primary prevention programs effectively in schools, and some programs are especially practical for use in schools. However, indiscriminant implementation without careful attention to the planning process will only result in failure and increased resistance to prevention efforts. Careful planning of modest prevention projects will have beneficial long-term results.

References

Allen, G., Chinsky, J., Larcen, S., Lochman, J., & Selinger, H. (1976). *Community psychology and the schools: A behaviorally oriented multilevel preventive approach.* Hillsdale, NJ: Erlbaum.

Alpert, J. L. (1983, August). *Future, prevention, change, and school psychology.* Presidential Address to Division 16 of the American Psychological Association at the Annual Convention, Anaheim, CA.

Barker, R. G., & Gump, P. (1964). *Big school, small school.* Stanford, CA: Stanford University Press.

Bower, E. M. (1964). The modification, mediation, and utilization of stress during the school years. *American Journal of Orthopsychiatry, 34,* 667-674.

Camp, B. W., & Bash, M. A. (1981). *Think aloud: Increasing social and cognitive skills—a problem-solving program for children.* Champaign, IL: Research Press.

Cowen, E. L. (1977). Baby steps toward primary prevention. *American Journal of Community Psychology, 5,* 1-22.

Cowen, E. L. (1980). The primary health project: Yesterday, today and tomorrow. *The Journal of Special Education, 14,* 133-154.

Cowen, E. L. (1984). A general structure model for primary prevention program development in mental health. *The Personnel and Guidance Journal, 62,* 485-490.

Cowen, E. L., Gesten, E. L., & Wilson, A. B. (1979). The primary mental health project (PMHP): Evaluation of current program effectiveness. *American Journal of Community Psychology, 7,* 293-303.

Elardo, P. T., & Cooper, M. (1977). *Project AWARE: A handbook for teachers.* Reading, MA: Addison-Wesley.

Felner, R. D., Ginter, M., & Primavera, J. (1982). Primary prevention during school transitions: Social support and environmental structure. *American Journal of Community Psychology, 10,* 277-290.

Gesten, E. L., De Apodaca, R. F., Rains, M., Weissberg, R. P., & Cowen, E. L. (1979). Promoting peer-related social competence in schools. In M. W. Kent & J. E. Rolf (Eds.), *Primary prevention of psychopathology. Volume 3: Social competence in children* (pp. 220-247). Hanover, NH: University Press of New England.

Hagin, R. A. (1980, September). *Prediction, prevention, presumption.* Distinguished Service Award Address presented at the Annual Meetings of the American Psychological Association, Montreal, Quebec, Canada.

Hauser-Cram, P. & Pierson, D. E. (1981). *The BEEP prekindergarten curriculum: A working paper.* Brookline, MA: Brookline Early Education Project.

Hohmann, M., Banet, B., & Weikart, D. P. (1979). *Young children in action: A manual for preschool educators.* Ypsilanti, MI: High/Scope Press.

Hyman, I. A. (1971). *Sensitivity training as a component of a parallel system to initiate educational change.* Paper presented at the 79th annual meetings of the American Psychological Association, Washington, DC.

Johnson, D. W., & Johnson, R. (1980). Promoting constructive student-student relationships through cooperative learning. In M. R. Reynolds & R. Bentz (Eds.), *Extending the challenge: Working toward a common body of practice for teachers.* Minneapolis, MN: National Support Systems Project, University of Minnesota.

Lazar, I., Darlington, R., & associates. (1982). Lasting effects of early education: A report from the consortium for longitudinal studies. *Society for Research in Child Development, 47,* 1-151.

Lorion, R. P. (1983). Evaluating preventive interventions: Guidelines for the serious social change agent. In R. D. Felner, L. Jason, J. Moritsugu, & S. S. Farber (Eds.), *Preventive psychology: Theory, research, and practice in community interventions* (pp. 252-268). New York: Pergamon.

Lorion, R. P., Work, W. C., & Hightower, A. D. (1984). A school-based multilevel preventive intervention: Issues in program development and evaluation. *The Personnel and Guidance Journal, 62,* 479-484.

Meyers, J., Parsons, R. D., & Martin, R. (1979). *Mental health consultation in the schools.* San Francisco: Jossey-Bass.

Moos, R. H. (1973). Conceptualization of human environments. *American Psychologist, 28,* 652-665.

Moos, R. H. (1974a). *The social climate scales: An overview.* Palo Alto, CA: Consulting Psychologists Press.

Moos, R. H. (1974b). *Evaluating treatment environments: A social ecological approach.* New York: John Wiley.

Moos, R. H. (1979). *Evaluating educational environments.* San Francisco: Jossey-Bass.

Ojemann, R. H. (1969). Incorporating psychological concepts in the school curriculum. In H. P. Clarizio (Ed.), *Mental health and the educative process.* Chicago: Rand-McNally.

Parsons, R. D., & Meyers, J. (1984). *Developing consultation skills.* San Francisco: Jossey-Bass

Pierson, D. E., Walker, D. K. & Tivnan, T. (1984). A school-based program from infancy to kindergarten for children and their parents. *Personnel and Guidance Journal 62,* 448-455.

Sarason, S. B. (1971). *The culture of the school and the problem of change.* Boston: Allyn & Bacon.

Shure, M. B., & Spivack, G. (1974). *A mental health program for kindergarten children: Training script.* Philadelphia: Department of Mental Health Sciences, Hahnemann University.

Shure, M. B., & Spivack, G. (1978). *Problem solving techniques in childrearing.* San Francisco: Jossey-Bass.

Shure, M. B., & Spivack, G. (1979). Interpersonal problem solving thinking and adjustment. In M. W. Kent & J. E. Rolf (Eds.), *Primary prevention of psychopathology: Volume III. Social competence in children.* Hanover, NH: University Press of New England.

Spivack, G., Platt, J. J., & Shure, M. B. (1976). *The problem solving approach to adjustment.* San Francisco: Jossey-Bass.

Spivack, G., & Shure, M. B. (1974). *Social adjustment of young children: A cognitive approach to solving real-life problems.* San Francisco: Jossey-Bass.

Stone, N., Pendleton, V., & Vaill, M. (1980). *Head start child and family mental health field specialist manual.* Contract #HEW (HHR) 105-77-1059. Washington, DC: Planning and Human Systems.

Weber, C. U., Foster, P. S., & Weikart, D. P. (1978). *An economic analysis of the Ypsilanti Perry Preschool Project: Monograph of the High/Scope Educational Research Foundation (Number Five).* Ypsilanti, MI: High/Scope Press.

Weikart, D. (1984). *Early childhood education: Lessons for the prevention of mental health problems in children.* Address presented to the 4th Annual Delaware Valley Conference on the Future of Psychology in the Schools. Sponsored by the Department of School Psychology, Temple University, Philadelphia.

Yurchak, M.J.H. (1975). *Infant-toddler curriculum of the Brookline early education project.* Brookline, MA: Brookline Early Education Project.

Chapter 6

SELF-HELP AND PREVENTION

ALFRED H. KATZ and JARED HERMALIN

This chapter has several purposes. First, to examine the concept of prevention, developed in public health; second, to consider the present roles, structure, and functions of self-help groups as a social resource for needy persons; third, to discuss a number of areas of human problems in which self-help groups are of actual or potential preventive significance; and fourth, to highlight the steps in self-help group development.

I. THE PUBLIC HEALTH CONCEPT OF PREVENTION

Prevention, of course, is a basic and multidimensional element of health care. However, it has been and continues to be strikingly neglected in clinical medicine. As Colombotos (1976) has pointed out, "The practice of medicine in this country is oriented toward the diagnosis and treatment of disease rather than toward its prevention. This orientation is reflected in how the overall health care system is organized, and in its *incentives* (e.g., how practitioners are reimbursed for their services). On the level of the individual physician, it is reflected in the great professional satisfaction and stimulation he or she derives

Authors' Note: The first seven sections of this chapter were written by the first author. The second author wrote the remaining sections.

from curative activities, rather than from preventive endeavors, and his or her perception of the greater medical value of the former.'' Because physicians are so central to the operations of the health care delivery system, it should not be surprising that the system, in fact, is a disease care delivery system. There is, however, an alternative paradigm developed in public health activities that helps to illuminate the concept and guide its applications. Along with the investigative tools of epidemiology and biostatistics, the public health formulations of prevention are particularly pertinent to the organization of programs for mass health improvement.

The notion of prevention emerged in public health sometime around the turn of the twentieth century, when there was special concern about the control of infectious diseases. A terminology was adopted and methods were developed to define the various steps necessary to mount programs that would control and subsequently eliminate communicable diseases. In less than a century, the following of these approaches has brought about some notable achievements. Infectious diseases that have been largely or totally eliminated include tuberculosis, smallpox, cholera, malaria, and poliomyelitis. These successes are attributable not only to the scientific advances made in the laboratories but also to the public health methods and programs that made it possible to apply such knowledge to the actual relief of human suffering.

The public health concept distinguishes three levels of prevention, usually referred to as primary, secondary, and tertiary prevention. *Primary prevention* means preventing what we know how to prevent. If a disease can be attributed to a viral or bacterial source, or to an environmental toxin, then the effects of that organism or agent can be controlled through environmental clean-up or by minimizing individual susceptibility through immunization and vaccination.

Secondary prevention in public health means finding and treating individuals with illnesses the effects of which we know how to terminate, arrest, or mitigate. This level thus involves a combination of early case-finding before a disease has become strongly manifest, and the application of corrective or remedial measures to individuals. These measures may not wipe out but will lessen, that is, in a weaker sense, "prevent" the further spread or worsening of the illness.

Tertiary prevention means limiting the disabilities an individual suffers from illness, once it has become clearly manifest. An example from mental illness is appropriate—the case of schizophrenia. At present, it is not known how to prevent any of the varieties of schizophrenia. However, at the secondary level of prevention, case-finding methods can be used to bring people into early remedial or supportive treatment; and in the tertiary level, social resources provided to sufferers will limit or reduce their individual disabilities in functioning, and thus "prevent" their further physical and psychosocial deterioration.

Thus, to sum up the public health approach, primary prevention means thwarting disease before it occurs. Secondary prevention means finding unapparent disease and treating it early. Tertiary prevention means effectively treating apparent disease to prevent serious later complications.

II. SELF-HELP GROUPS

Let us now review some findings about the status and nature of self-help groups in modern societies. The last 20 years have witnessed a striking increase in the formation of various kinds of self-help groups in Western countries. Their growth has been so rapid and dynamic that they are difficult to count and classify. Current data are fragmentary. My estimate (Katz & Bender, 1976) that there were as early as 1976 some half million separate self-help groups in North America, embracing five to ten million member participants, was probably conservative at the time and is now certainly outmoded. That estimate was based on listings of more than 500 national organizations, each including local units; the latter ranging in number from a mere handful to the 27,000 chapters of Alcoholics Anonymous. The proliferation of self-help groups is not confined to those with national affiliations. The number of ad hoc local groups is immense. My 1976 estimate included the speculation that at least 40,000-50,000 unaffiliated local self-help organizations could be found, in addition to many state and regional organizations. Indeed, every community in the United States and Canada with a population of 20,000 or more probably has at least a few local or nationally affiliated self-help groups, and many are in process of organization, perhaps averaging a growth rate of 5 to 10 new groups daily. Although less populous than the United States, and not having all the same pressures toward the creation of such groups, other Western countries have also experienced a rapid growth of self-help organizations in the past two decades. In the United Kingdom, Robinson and Henry (1978) have identified hundreds of self-help groups, both national and local. Van Harberden and Lafaille (1978) have published a similar account of the situation in Holland. Australia and South America have extensive arrays of such groups and they are also known to exist in some countries of Eastern Europe, such as Poland and Yugoslavia.

Contemporary groups embracing the self-help principles and practices include (a) the natural and informal social networks of family, workmates, schoolmates, neighbors, friends, and peers, and (b) a wide range of largely self-organized and self-directing healing, educational, economic, and socially supporting groups. Self-help forms and practices are found in a variety of organizations that promote care in physical and mental health for the self or relatives, in housing cooperatives and other economic projects, in groups set up to help so-called deviants, (for example, homosexuals, ex-convicts, former mental patients, and ex-prostitutes). Groups exist for single parents, for the parents of runaway children, the parents of gifted children, parents with actual or potential problems of child abuse and child neglect, parents of gay children, couples choosing childlessness, and so on. In the health field there are groups for nearly all of the 200 major diseases listed by the World Health Organization, from anorexia nervosa to von Willibrandt's disease. There are many antidrug organizations that exist as well as a number that combat compulsive gambling. There are ex-prisoner organizations with differing ideologies and programs. In mental health there are a legion of groups for specified diagnostic categories—neurosis, schizoprenia, manic-depressive syndrome, as well as for more general mental problems. An exhaustive catalog of these proliferating groups in the broad health and welfare field cannot be made because they are growing so rapidly and changing so quickly that they outstrip the tempo of present resources for data collection.

III. DEFINITION OF SELF-HELP GROUPS

The half-million or more separate self-help organizations embody an extraordinary variety of types, purposes, structures, and ideological features, tap a variety of motives, and appeal to a vast range of members. To bring scientific order into this domain, through definitions and taxonomies, is a difficult task.

Approaches to definition have attempted first to define the nature and distinctive properties of the groups. A number of such definitions have been formulated since the mid-1970s, of which the most widely cited and used is that of Katz and Bender (1976):

> Self-help groups are voluntary, small group structures for mutual aid and the accomplishment of a special purpose. They are usually formed by peers who have come together for mutual assistance in satisfying a common need, overcoming a common handicap or life-disrupting problem, and bringing about desired social and/or personal change. The initiators and members of such groups perceive that their needs are not, or cannot be, met by or through existing social institutions. Self-help groups emphasize face-to-face social interactions and the assumption of personal responsibility by members. They often provide material assistance, as well as emotional support; they are frequently "cause"-oriented, and promulgate any ideology or values through which members may attain an enhanced sense of personal identity.

To this definition, its authors appended a further list of defining attributes as follows: "(1) Self-help groups always involve face-to-face interactions. (2) The origin of self-help groups is spontaneous (they are not usually set-up by an outside group). (3) Personal participation is an extremely important ingredient; bureaucratization is antithetical to the self-help organization. (4) The members agree on and engage in some actions. (5) Typically, the groups start from a condition of powerlessness. (6) The groups fill needs for a reference group, a point of connection and identification with others, a base for activity and a source of ego-reinforcement.''

By these attributes, then, self-help groups may be distinguished from ''mutual aid'' groupings and agreements among those who exercise political or economical power—such as unions, cartels, corporation boards, ''old boy'' networks, and friendship cliques. The groups are distinguished also from various voluntary membership organizations, such as ''Service organizations,'' oriented to traditional philanthropy (the Elks, Shriners) or public education (League of Women Voters). The definition also excludes such temporary or uncalculated natural associations as children playing together, the short-lived ''emergency col-lectivism'' of neighbors in times of natural disasters, and ''encounter groups.'' All of these usually lack a common problem, a special purpose, or an ideology, and they are all usually transient.

The above definition of self-help groups emphasizes that the group, whatever its origin, belongs to and is run by its members. *Autonomy* is thus a key functional characteristic of the self-help group; that is, self-direction from within by members, rather than direction by outsiders, for example professionals.

IV. A THEORETICAL BACKGROUND FOR SELF-HELP EFFECTIVENESS

Let us now look at some findings and theoretical interpreta-tions of the actual and potential significance of self-help groups in prevention of disease and the maintenance of health. It has been clear for some time that the chief problems affecting the health of populations in advanced countries are the chronic diseases, which account for some 75% or 80% of current morbidity and mortality. It is also clear that personal behavior, as summed up in the term "lifestyle," is highly involved, in interaction with the physical and social environment in both the causation and management of such chronic long-term diseases or conditions. The examples of coronary artery disease, cancer, and hypertension are familiar in this respect. From many studies of ill populations, a further important general finding has emerged regarding vulnerability, namely, that persons who lack stable and satisfying social supports, that is, those who are isolated, have the highest risk of morbidity and mortality in the major conditions.

The rates of illness and death in a given population seem to vary more according to the degree of social support and interactions than to the presence or absence of any particular hazard or behavior, such as smoking or obesity. Being vulnerable or at-risk also correlates highly with the nature of one's self-concept, in particular with the individual's sense of being in control of his or her life and the factors that affect it. A positive self-image, including a sense of one's ability to master the environment and to cope with life pressures, seems correlated with the tendency to resist illness, and, conversely, in its absence, to succumb to those pressures. As a corollary to this finding, epidemiologic studies have also indicated that persons who are in relatively weaker, subordinate, or powerless positions in any population group stand the greatest risk of falling ill and have the poorest prognosis for recovery and rehabilitation.

This view of the importance of social supports in health and disease was succinctly presented by one of the leading social epidemiologists of the past quarter century, the late John Cassel of the University of North Carolina School of Public Health. One of Cassel's last papers summarizes beliefs he had come to from his own research and his extensive knowledge of the work of others.

Reviewing many studies, Cassel (1976, p. 110) wrote, "A remarkably similar set of social circumstances characterizes people who develop tuberculosis and schizophrenia, become alcoholics, are victims of multiple accidents, or commit suicide.

Common to all these people is a marginal status in society. They are individuals who for a variety of reasons (ethnic minorities rejected by the dominant majority in their neighborhood; high sustained rates of residential and occupational mobility; broken homes or isolated living circumstances) have been deprived of meaningful social contact.'' He went on, ''The existing data have led me to believe that we should no longer treat psychosocial processes as unidimensional stressors or non-stressors, but rather as two-dimensional, one category being stressors, and another being protective or beneficial. . . the property common to these processes is the strength of the social supports provided by the primary groups of most importance to the individual'' (pp. 111-112).

Cassel (1976, p. 121) concluded his review with recommendations that embody the use of self-help approaches: ''With advancing knowledge, it is perhaps not too far-reaching to imagine a preventive health service in which professionals are involved largely in the diagnostic aspects—identifying families and groups at high risk by virtue of their lack of fit with their social milieu and determining the particular nature and form of the social supports that can and should be strengthened if such people are to be protected from disease outcomes. The intervention actions then could well be undertaken by nonprofessionals, provided that adequate guidance and specific direction were given.''

V. HELPING NETWORKS AND PREVENTION

The research findings on which Cassel's views were based have been supplemented and reinforced by more recent work.

Researchers concerned with factors that help individuals cope with stress are increasingly focusing on social support. Individuals suffering from malignant disease, physical disability, death of a close friend or family member, rape, and job loss have all been found to adjust better when they receive social support (Caplan, 1979). For example, Gore (1978) found that unemployed men who felt unsupported had more symptoms of illness and were more depressed than unemployed men who felt supported. High levels of depression are frequently found for individuals with low levels of social support. Berkman and Syme (1979), in a prospective study, found that people who lacked social ties had higher mortality rates than did those with social ties.

As Cassel suggested, these data offer clues to a methodology of prevention that has not been formerly appreciated. Prevention is not simply a matter of giving people didactic instruction on personal health habits, the right foods to eat, exercise, sleep, and so on, nor is it simply a matter of multiphasic screening or having periodic health examinations by health professionals. As Cassel (1976, p. 121) stated, "Disease, with rare exceptions, has not been prevented by finding and treating sick individuals, but by modifying those environmental factors which facilitate its occurrence."

Prevention at the primary level of both physical/mental illness thus is correlated with improving how people feel about themselves; one available way of achieving such primary improvement is to enhance their social ties and connections. In the mental health field, these ideas have received expression in the Report of the President's Commission on Mental Health (1978), as well as in the Reports of the White House Conference on Handicapped Individuals (1977).

A few paragraphs from the Mental Health Commission's report (1978, pp. 166-167) give some flavor of that group's thinking regarding the importance of community support approaches as a component in professional knowledge and actions:

> *Naturally occurring helping networks exist independently of professional caregivers and formal caregiving institutions.* [emphasis added] Often they are invisible to professional scrutiny because the assistance given and received is qualitatively different from that offered within disciplinary frames of reference and is rendered outside the structure of the human services agencies within which most professionals work, i.e., within the family; in kin, kith, friendship and neighborhood social networks;

religious denominations; common interest and mutual help groups. Professionals need to affirm the existence and worth of these natural helping networks. *Linkages need to be developed between these social and community support systems, including mutual help groups, and the professional and formal institutional caregiving systems.* They should be established on a basis of cooperation and collaboration, not cooptation and control, and without disturbing the potency of their very different helping processes. These linkages can provide people in need of help individual choice and freedom of movement between natural and formal systems of care. They can promote professionally responsive and consumer-accountable services.

Particularly, then, when applied to persons suffering from chronic illness, unrelieved social tensions, sheer lonliness, and the absence of social connections, self-help groups may be viewed as supplying the vital elements of social support when these are otherwise lacking. In this sense, the groups can function as quasi- or substitute families. Furthermore, as the experience of the last 25 years has also shown, they also aid members and participants in attaining a firmer and more positive self-image through various means, such as redefining and reducing the stigmatizing effects of the problem, overcoming the individual's or family's sense of isolation (the belief that they are the only ones affected), and emphasizing activities that patients and their families can engage in themselves without prolonged dependence on professionals. The latter benefits occurring after the establishment of illness/ disability may be conceptualized as examples of secondary and tertiary prevention a la the public health model.

VI. SELF-HELP GROUPS AND COMMON HUMAN TRANSITIONS AND CRISES

Having briefly sketched a general theoretical explanation for the significance and functioning of self-help group participation in human populations, let us now discuss their prevention possibilities in relation to some common personal and family crises. These will be presented broadly in relation to chronological stages of the life-history of individuals and families.

Perinatal Health Care

Perinatal is defined as the period between conception and one year of life. Whereas self-help groups such as A.A., Recovery, Inc., and Make Today Count are familiar and highly publicized, not so well-known are groups that deal with perinatal issues— such as infertility, childbirth education, caesarean deliveries, prematurity, neonatal death, breast-feeding, child-abuse, terminal illness, and genetic and other handicapping and chronic illness in young children. There are self-help groups that specialize in helping parents meet each of these serious problems and needs. Childbirth education groups on a self-help basis prepare couples for the entire gestational, labor, and delivery period. Couples are made aware of their options in childbirth, and through interactions on a self-help-group basis are helped to define more clearly available choices that will be satisfactory to them.

To quote from a recent paper on self-help resources for parents in the perinatal period:

> Parents Anonymous and Parents United have been helpful for parents involved in child abuse and neglect. Other parent groups have formed due to a child with a handicap; e.g., spina bifida, cleft palate, Down's Syndrome, autism, etc. Individuals facing infertility or couples considering adoption have also joined together to provide mutual support and assistance. Crisis events such as the death of an infant or a very young child have led to the development of groups such as Compassionate Friends, Candlelighters & AMEND (AID to Mothers Experiencing Neo-natal Death).

> In some instances, perinatal self-help approaches have expanded beyond group meetings to the development of hotlines, visitor programs and peer counseling or parent resource systems. Several Newborn Intensive Care Units (NB ICU's) utilize "graduate" parents to offer lay counseling to parents of critically ill infants. Groups like Parents of SIDS (Sudden Infant Death Syndrome) and Empty Cradle (fetal and newborn loss) provide both hotlines and one-on-one resource parents to aid the newly-bereaved. (Bryant, 1983)

Clinicians testify that all of these kinds of self-help groups for families experiencing a crisis around reproductive behavior or childbirth perform significant functions at all levels of prevention. It is clear that the groups for parents who have a child born with or acquiring a disabling disease or condition can be benefical in both the cognitive and affective areas in preventing further physical and mental health problems.

Much recent research has emphasized the importance of early bonding between the mother and the newborn as a key factor in the infant's emotional and cognitive development, and in the mother's parenting abilities. With prematures, who may spend days, weeks, or months in an intensive care unit (ICU), normal bonding is delayed, and is much more difficult to achieve after the infant's discharge. A study by Minde et al. (1975) showed that participants in a mother's self-help group visited their infants in the ICU more frequently, interacted with them more during visits, and felt more competent about their subsequent parenting role than did nonparticipants. Such self-help participation may be viewed as a factor in primary prevention of possible later pathology in the child and the family.

The incidence of caesarean delivery has shown a steady increase in recent years. A poor caesarean birth experience can also have negative effects on the mother's mental health, and thus on her parenting abilities and the familial environment during the postnatal period and later. Caesarean support groups on the self-help model have been shown to provide "a safe atmosphere in which women can share their concern without fear of being misunderstood or belittled" (Lipson, 1982).

Parents who experience the death of their infant through miscarriage, stillbirth, or other causes need support, understanding, and information to assist them in their grief. Such self-help groups as Empty Cradle, AMEND, and The Compassionate Friends (loss of a child at any age) assist such parents through open and frank group discussion, provision of one-on-one peer counseling, overcoming feelings of isolation in their grief, and so on. That these resources can help prevent later pathologies that may arise from lack of resources for working through the grief process seems clear.

Children with a Handicap

With families where a child with a physical/mental anomaly, disorder, or defect has been born, there is usually a need to come to terms with such emotional reactions as grief, self-blame, and rejection of the child; to work through an often profound family crisis before healthy, supportive parenting styles and a nurturant family environment can be established. Even in the absence of prolonged parental/emotional distress, the parenting of a child with special problems presents many difficulties. Material needs and psychological dilemmas abound—for example, finances, medical care, schooling, housing adaptations, baby-sitting and other respite care; uncertainty about developmental expectations, discipline, and handling—that is, walking the narrow line between necessary physical cautions and overprotectiveness; avoidance of the inculcation of prolonged dependency and a negative self-image in the child. These and many related issues require strength, consistency, and sharing and agreement between the parents. Without these positive elements in the family setting, pathological psychosocial reactions can be expected in both the child and parents. Many clinicians have recognized the dangers to the successful growth and social maturation of the child and to the integrity of the family unit if these elements of constructive behavior and attitude are not present or promoted. Most of the recommendations for preventing pathological interactions and dysfunctions in these families and their children involve professional/clinical interventions.

But the use of parent self-help groups constitutes an alternative, sometimes more effective resource and coping strategy. Some 30 years ago, in my doctoral study, published in summary form as "Parents of the Handicapped," (Katz, 1961), I cited evidence from my interviews with parents of children suffering from cerebral palsy, mental retardation, muscular dystrophy, and schizophrenia of the manifold benefits the parents derived from participation in self-help groups for these disorders. Since that time, a host of clinical and empirical studies of self-help-group support activities in a wide array of child health problems have come into the literature, and provide confirmation of these early findings.

The assistance gained by parents from participation in self-help groups can not only be considered as a primary preventive of family dysfunctioning and its consequences, but is significant also in the psychosocial development and the prevention of further physical/mental problems in the child. In recent years, much clinical work and research has highlighted the importance of parent stimulation of infants and young children suffering from central nervous system disorders and developmental deficits. An excellent example of parent participation may be cited from the Down's Syndrome project at the University of Washington.

> The staff from the first encourage the parents to interact with the infant constantly during his waking hours: to cuddle, to talk to, to hold, and to play with the infant. And, at first, parents are often astounded as they watch the staff doing all of those things. But the staff have found that their enthusiasm about the baby is contagious—parents who had earlier been somehow frightened of this infant with his "differences" could begin to react to him as they might automatically have reacted to a normal infant....

> Parents are involved from the moment their child is seen by our staff and then throughout his school program. They are trained to use at home many of the exercise and instructional procedures used at school. When their children reach preschool age, they work in the classrooms—they are trained to be observers, data-takers, and teaching assistants. They use many of the data-taking procedures at home so that they and the staff can determine whether the child's behaviors at home and at school are complementing each other, and can then make informed decisions together about his behavioral objectives and program.

> Parents attend staff meetings on days they have worked in school; they have individual and group conferences with their children's teachers at frequent intervals—if necessary, by telephone....

> The parents' activities in the larger community are formidable. Some serve as counselors; they are on call at several Seattle hospitals to visit and talk to parents of newborn Down's syndrome infants almost as soon as the new parents have been told about their child's diagnosis. They lecture to students in

various University of Washington departments—education, psychology, social work, and in the School of Medicine. Several have written articles for Sharing Our Caring, a nationally distributed journal specifically concerned with Down's syndrome. Finally, in what is surely one of the most appropriate testimonials to "parents as partners," several young couples who have moved beyond commuting distance... have been able, on the basis of their training here, to organize and maintain preschool programs for young handicapped children in communities where previously there had been no educational opportunities for this population. (Hayden & Haring, 1976)

It is clear that parent participation in such stimulation programs is reinforced when the parents join with other parents in a mutual aid group, which thus may be viewed as a potent resource for prevention at the secondary level.

The learning of self-management skills by children suffering from some chronic diseases is also facilitated by child and parent involvement in group education activities. Young hemophiliacs now routinely do their own venipunctures, learning to inject prophylactic materials that minimize the occurrence of internal hemorrhages, and thus reduce the incidence of crippling arthropathies (Jones, 1982). Young asthma patients learn to monitor their breathing capacities, to recognize impending airway obstructions, and to take remedial actions. Such secondary prevention programs, involving the active co-operation of child and parents, have proliferated widely in many chronic disorders, and are clearly pertinent to secondary and tertiary prevention. Self-help groups often organize this kind of program or support those organized by professionals.

Later Problems of Childhood-Adolescence

When it comes to problems that frequently arise later in a child's development, self-help groups also can play important roles in primary and secondary prevention. Common problems in latency, puberty, and adolescence include difficulties in child/parent relationships, eating disorders, substance abuse, establishment of sexual identity, and school alienation and drop-out.

In adolescence, problems of identity establishment, dependency-independence conflicts, vocational choice and preparation, and sexuality come to the fore. Failure to solve or resolve these pervasive problems is predictive of much adolescent pathology of a behavioral character.

Teenage "rap" groups organized on the self-help model embody the well-known peer communication preference of adolescents, and have demonstrated that they can be influential toward healthy teen social values and functioning (Hayden & Haring, 1976). In particular, programs for overcoming adolescent drug abuse, alcoholism, sexually transmitted diseases, and teenage pregnancy have and continue to rely heavily on self-help approaches, which are demonstrably the "treatment of choice" in such conditions. (Creer, 1978).

Self-help groups have also been effective with respect to the employment situation of young people. Vocational choice, the development of a "working personality," which includes the self-concept, attitudes toward supervision and authority, work habits, and so on, have all been fostered by specific self-help groups.

For young people who have a physical/mental disability or handicap, the Centers for Independent Living, which in the past 10 years have had an extensive growth in many urban centers, provide job counseling and placement skills in self-presentation to potential employers—all by using the self-help group discussion method.

Problems of Adult Life

These are of course protean factors encompassing work, family and other social relationships, migration and mobility, changes in values and lifestyle, and so on. We cannot discuss the problems encountered and resources needed when individuals confront disrupting conditions in all of these areas, but, echoing Freud's well-known formula, two can be singled out: disruptions in the work situation and in family relationships.

Economic changes of recent years have altered familiar concepts and expectations of full employment and job stability. Unemployment in double-digit figures, displacement of workers in industries previously thought inalterable components of the economy, the shifts toward automation, high-technology and service occupations, the geographic relocations of industries from traditional to newer areas such as the Sunbelt states—all have resulted and continue to result in major stresses in the U.S. occupational force. There is ample documentation of the serious effects on the physical/mental health status of affected workers and their families. (Caplan, 1979).

Coping with the material and psychological effects of these change-producing stresses often is beyond the abilities of individual workers and families, and poses a challenge in the prevention of physical/mental disorders in this at-risk population. Among various approaches to these problems, the use of self-help organizations and techniques for displaced workers has shown promise. In California, with the cooperation of the State Departments of Mental Health and Employment and Development, and the companies and unions involved, special retraining programs have been mounted, in the northern and southern parts of the state, to assist workers from automobile plants that have been closed or relocated to other states. In addition to vocational assessment training and placement for other occupations, the programs include monitoring of the physical and mental health of displaced workers and their families and both one-on-one and group counseling. Self-help groups of workers and their spouses have been organized in these programs to promote cooperation around material needs such as food, but also to make possible the expression of personal feelings and attitudes about the job loss, necessary adaptations in terms of personal and family attitudes and roles, support and reinforcement for undergoing shifts in career expectations, retraining, relocation, and so on. Preliminary data from these demonstration projects reveal that participants in the self-help groups have fewer physical/mental problems and are able to accomplish occupational role and family relationship changes more expeditiously and effectively than nonparticipants (Creer, 1978).

In 1981, the Alcohol, Drug Abuse and Mental Health Administration (ADAMHA) of the U.S. Department of Health &

Human Services held a conference on Health Promotion/Prevention at the Worksite. This conference discussed various methods for reducing employee stress, including work environment modification and Employee Assistance Programs, and it called attention to a hitherto "untapped resource"—employee support groups on the self-help model. It was emphasized that such groups provide an effective opportunity to discuss not only worksite stresses but other worker problems, such as family relationship, child-rearing, lifestyles, and so on (Costello, 1976).

Family relationships have proved to be one of the important subject areas around which many self-help groups have come into being. Divorce, separation, single parenthood, bereavement, child-rearing, the situation of adoptees and their adoptive and biological parents, child abuse/neglect, and other kinds of family violence are all important social traumas that create short- or longer-term crises and stresses for the individuals and family units experiencing them, who are thus at risk of depression and other undesirable sequelae. Self-help groups exist in increasing numbers and variety to assist individuals and family units in coping with and surmounting such traumas, and thus can play a significant role in the prevention of serious disorders.

Retirement and Problems of Elder Citizens

With demographic changes resulting from bio-medical and social advances that have brought about increases in life expectancy and reductions in mortality/morbidity, the problems of elderly and aging citizens come to the forefront of national attention.

In general, the elderly have an increased risk of incurring chronic disease and disability; they also stand at the greatest risk of social isolation and dependency through retirement, and the loss or absence of meaningful activities and connections with others.

In discussing this subject, it is important not to conform to common stereotypes by considering all persons over 65 (or 60) as a homogeneous population, but to differentiate various groups among them, for whom both distinctive problems and various possibilities of self-help may exist and be appropriate. Four groups should be distinguished: the well-aged, who are basically independent and as fully functional as any segment of the population; the aged who have one or more chronic health problems, but are not significantly limited or disabled in their functioning; the aged having chronic conditions that are severely limiting—for example, those who are homebound; and, last, the so-called frail elderly, aged 75 or more, many of whom are in nursing homes or other institutions. The mix of problems encountered, of possible activities, of useful knowledge and skills, of involvement of relatives, and of possible participation in self-help groups is clearly different for each of the above groups.

In a review of self-care and self-help programs for the elderly, Robert Butler (1979/1980), former director of the National Institute on Aging, concludes with the following statement:

> Self-care and self-help, propelled by a variety of social forces, are moving to prominence on the health care scene. While their roles are not yet clearly defined, they show great promise. It seems only reasonable that this potential be tapped to benefit the elderly: the ailing, who must cope with disability and chronic disease; the isolated, who can join in shared experiences; the stultified, who can discover new ideas and pleasures; the impoverished, who can participate without paying; the bewildered, who can be guided by their peers; the grieving, who can better adjust to their losses; the retired, who have new leisure to learn about and take better care of their bodies.

In addition to self-help groups that organize around health problems of the elderly themselves, it is important to note the many self-help groups that have been formed by those—usually relatives—who are caretakers for elderly persons who suffer from debilitating diseases. Thus, as more has become known about Alzheimer's as a clinical entity, self-help groups for Alzheimer's disease have recently sprung up in a number of localities; the disease clearly poses severe problems to family members. Huntington's Disease, for which there are several national organizations in the United States made up of relatives and sufferers organized on a self-help basis, is another example that should be included in an account of self-help organizations to meet problems of the elderly.

Perhaps the most rapidly growing self-help group of the past decade is the National Alliance of the Mentally Ill, which is a federation of many local, state, and regional associations of mental patients, their relatives, and friends set up in 1979. The NAMI now numbers some 30,000 members in 90 groups in 48 states, and maintains a legislative office in Washington, D.C. A major stimulus to its dynamic growth has been the deinstitutionalization of mental patients, which has obviously brought many "chronic" schizophrenics and other psychotic patients back to families and communities ill-equipped to take care of them. It seems evident that many of the returned "chronic" patients had spent years in mental hospitals, and would be in older age groups. As a self-help consumer group, NAMI is concerned with strengthening the family as a support system, "issues of stigma and misinformation," research, needed changes in treatment and service delivery, and with the maintenance of adequate funding for federal and state programs for the mentally ill. The importance of such activities to all levels of prevention, both for social policy and programs, and for individual patients and their families, seems clearly evident.

VII. SOME COMMON UNDERLYING PROCESSES

Having briefly surveyed the pertinence to prevention of participation in self-help groups and other social support systems, at various stages of the life cycle, it is now important to analyze some common elements embodied in such participation, despite the diversity of both the human problems dealt with and the particularities of the support groups themselves.

Three common aspects of self-help groups will be discussed: (1) their process of empowerment, (2) their process of role modeling, and (3) the effects of their action-orientation.

The broadest underlying common property of such groups is that they foster *empowerment*—that is, they facilitate the individual's sense of power or mastery over the predictable and unforeseen stresses and trauma of social living. The widower, the adult who loses a job, the parents of a child who has died— all experience hardship; these traumatic situations impose stresses that often exceed the lone individual's or family's coping resources, and that, if prolonged and not resolved, can lead to pathological consequences. Empowerment means increasing the ability of individuals and families to cope with such stresses, and the process seems correlated with the strengths of the available social supports and the self-concept. Self-help groups thus often function as substitute or quasi-families that not only give material aid and emotional sustenance but also strengthen the individual's self-esteem and consequent feelings of power in being able to cope with disruptive events or environments.

Role modeling—the example of peers who encounter and overcome the same problems—is a powerful dynamic factor in the social learning arising from experience in mutual aid groups, and it is a factor not available from professional sources.

Bandura (1985), a leading social-learning theorist, summarizes the importance of social and role modeling:

> Virtually all learning phenomena resulting from direct experience occur on a vicarious basis by observing other people's behavior and its consequences for them. The capacity to learn by observation enables people to acquire roles and integrated patterns of behavior without having to form them gradually by tedious trial and error. The constraints of time, resources and mobility impose severe limits on the types of situations and activities that can be explored directly. Through social modeling people can draw on vast sources of information, exhibited and authored by others, for expanding their knowledge and skills.... Seeing modeling behavior succeed for others increases the tendency to behave in similar ways, whereas seeing behavior punished decreased like tendencies.

The third common aspect or attribute generally found in self-help groups may be termed *action-orientation*. This attribute is related to both empowerment and role modeling, but may be considered a later stage or a resultant of these two processes.

After greater self-confidence has been achieved, and in following the examples of role models in the group, the individual participant is encouraged to engage in actions that improve either his or her individual situation or that of the group as a whole. Encouragement of such behavioral changes in participants may be an explicit or implicit group objective.

Psychodynamic formulations analyze this process as anxiety-reducing because the participant's growing understanding of the problem leads to personal actions to prevent its recurrence or to mitigate its effects. Action is counterposed to mere passive discussion, which may reinforce or perpetuate anxiety.

The analysis that has been sketched above is closely akin to conceptualizations of Antonovsky (1979), a prominent medical sociologist. Antonovsky posits a "sense of coherence" in patients and potential patients as the sum or result of what he terms the individual's "generalized resistance resources" (GRRs). He sees the sense of coherence as closely correlated with, even determinative of the individual's health status. Generalized resistance resources are defined "as any characteristic of the person, the group or the environment that can facilitate tension management." Antonovsky (1979, p. 99) identifies three kinds of GRRs: "adaptability on the physiological, biochemical, psychological, cultural and social levels; profound ties to concrete immediate others; and commitment of and institutionalized ties between the individual and the total community."

The totality of these GRRs make up the sense of coherence that Antonovsky (1979, p. 123) conceives as "a global orientation that expresses the extent to which one has a pervasive enduring, though dynamic, feeling of confidence that one's internal and external environments are predictable and that there is a high probability that things will work out as well as can be reasonably expected."

Antonovsky's concept of coherence relates closely to that of empowerment that has been discussed. The sense of being able to control one's inner and outer environments is clearly a major component of one's self-esteem and self-confidence. Such a positive outlook correlates highly with Antonovsky's and Cassel's notion of "profound, concrete ties to immediate others" and with Cassel's views regarding resistance or vulnerability to stressors, and the avoidance or overcoming of pathological processes. These concepts illuminate the role of self-help groups in facilitating prevention at all three levels of the public health paradigm.

The application of such concepts in the planning of preventive activities in the universe of human service programs has been rarely consciously attended to or attempted. The concepts highlight the importance of recognizing, fostering, and consciously using informal support groups of all types, including self-help groups, as resources in aiding troubled people cope with life pressures and crises. Such support groups perform services of emotional and material sustenance, present peer models of successful coping, aid in the establishment of positive self-concepts through education and reinforcement in problem-solving and self-management skills, and provide opportunities for the open sharing of problems in a nonthreatening atmosphere. In all these aspects, and in major periods of the life cycle, they present conventional but underutilized, and easily-realized possibilities for the prevention of individual and social disease and distress.

VIII. DEVELOPMENT OF SELF-HELP GROUPS

Reasons for Developing New Groups

Although there are an extensive number of self-help groups currently in existence, they are not always accessible to the potential user. A specific problem-focused group, for example, may meet at an inconvenient time or be located across town, out of easy transportation reach. The group may be targeted to a particular audience (e.g., the patient), eliminating the participation of concerned significant others (spouse, parent, or other relative). Or membership may be so large as to permit each member only a very limited amount of time to discuss his or her problem.

Further, the philosophical orientation of the group may be at odds with one's own philosophy, making participation in the group uncomfortable and compromising. Indeed, the available self-help groups may not even address the specific concerns or issues that brought the person to the group in the first place, particularly if its focus is outer-directed (advocacy) versus inner-directed.

In instances where present self-help groups prove unsatisfactory, or in areas where there is a lack of specific types of self-help groups, the situation is ripe for the flowering of a new group. The process begins by the realization that there is a need to fill a gap in the service delivery model. Before embarking on the creation of a new group, however, the individual should examine whether unmet needs can be satisfied by any other currently existing system. This means that the individual should explore alternative facilities and programs. It is much easier to join an already existing operation than to start a new organization or group from scratch.

The desired self-help qualities shown in Table 6.1 should thus be sought in currently existing groups or programs.

Once it has become clear that other community alternatives are lacking in one or more of the above essential qualities, the individual may seriously raise the question of whether he or she wants to spend the necessary time developing a new group.

Characteristics of Self-Help Group Founders

Although the task of developing a self-help group can prove quite rewarding emotionally, not everyone is capable of starting a self-help group. A founder must be able to give affirmative responses to, at least, most of these key requirements (or be joined by one or more other persons able to fulfill such requirements). (See Table 6.2.)

In addition, many groups are founded and led by individuals sharing the problem or concern of other group members. Although this need not always be the case, it often does help to coalesce the group and provide the founder more credibility in the decision-making process.

Demographic variables, such as age, sex, race, religion, and socioeconomic status, are not usually considered to be the most

TABLE 6.1   Self-Help Qualities

(1) Nonclinical atmosphere
(2) Mutual support and encouragement
(3) Peer egalitarian structure
(4) Non-time-oriented membership
(5) Emphasis on face-to-face interaction
(6) Sense of group spirit/belonging
(7) Congruence of membership philosophical and action orientations
(8) Personal input into the decision-making process
(9) Minimization of membership fees and donations

TABLE 6.2   Founder Attributes

(1) Willingness to devote personal time to group formation
(2) Ability to network successfully with organizations, agencies, and groups to recruit membership/resources
(3) Skill in the development of flyers, brochures, and media announcements
(4) Ability to seek out and obtain a cost-effective meeting place
(5) Skill in group process development
(6) Ability to help the group define relevant goals, objectives, and action strategies
(7) Psychological capacity to be flexible and tolerant of a diversity of opinion
(8) Ability to take charge and act as facilitator, mediator, and arbiter (at least during the group's formative stages)
(9) Yet have the capacity to surrender control of the group as the group process evolves

important characteristics in a self-help group founder. The ability to mobilize a group around the stated concerns or problems is paramount.

The Recruitment Process

Following the decision to become a group founder, the next important order of business is to gain a membership. Many groups tend to average about 10-12 members. Others, such as Alcoholics Anonymous, can be much larger. It thus becomes imperative to decide on the number of members to be sought in the immediate future.

This resolution can be a function of several components: the amount of time to be expended; the ability to obtain lists of potential members from relevant health/mental health/social service facilities; coparticipation of one or more other individuals, groups, or agencies in recruiting membership; one's perceived ability to lead or manage a group of varying size; prevalence of potential members in the community; and the costs involved.

If three psychiatric centers each supplied the names of 10 candidates, development of a patient group would certainly be eased. Similarly, gaining a listing of 10 abused women from multiple resource services would certainly speed the development of an abused women's group.

Generally, however, names are not divulged to outside parties, for confidentiality purposes. In such instances, a variety of strategies may be employed: (a) The agency representative can disclose information about the support group to potential candidates. Each can then voluntarily choose (or not choose) to attend a group meeting, have their names divulged to the group founder, or get in touch with the founder directly; (b) pamphlets or brochures describing the group can be dis-seminated; or (c) notices can be circulated on community bulletin boards, with a reply telephone number. The more cooperation one is able to obtain from an agency dealing with the target audience, the quicker the recruitment process can be completed, all other things being equal.

It is also possible that despite desired group size, many more requests for membership might be received than originally desired.

HIGH MEMBERSHIP AVAILABILITY

If too many members are taken into the group, some founders feel that there is little time per meeting for each member to vent pent-up emotions as well as speak his or her peace. Enhanced membership can also elongate the decision-making process on specific items as well as lead to multiple factions. It is thus up to the founder in the early days of the group to determine how many members the group will tolerate initially. (Later on, of course, it becomes a group decision.)

Several alternatives are available. The easiest alternative is to accept all who apply. A second alternative is to limit membership to about 10-12 in the initial group and develop subsequent groups of about the same size. This alternative assumes that another founder or leader can be found for these additional groups. A single individual, unless employed to do so, is usually reluctant to start up more than a single group at any one time. A third alternative is to maintain the initial goal of 10-12 members and keep additional candidates on a waiting list until such time as the group feels comfortable enough to absorb new members. A fourth strategy is to contact professionals working in the area of group process (or more specifically, self-help) to see if they might be interested in starting a subsequent group. A fifth strategy is to contact self-help groups at the regional or national level to see if they would be willing to participate. Very often groups possess their own trainers and speakers and are willing to assist new chapters. Finally, a sixth alternative is to contact an areawide self-help clearinghouse (of which there are now about 20 across the country). They will either help to develop self-help groups directly (by utilizing their staff personnel in conjunction with the host) or will indirectly contribute through extensive consultation, either in person or via telephone or written materials. (Either author can be contacted for a listing of these self-help clearinghouses.)

In terms of recruiting members, we have thus far distinguished the positive side: cooperation from agencies, available resource listings of potential members, and a large response rate. But the opposite can also be true.

LOW MEMBERSHIP AVAILABILITY

In this situation the one or more founders of the group will have to concentrate efforts on securing members from the community at large. A sufficient cadre of potential members will not be immediately available from resource agencies.

Media Recruitment. Quite often recruitment strategy takes the form of publishing ads in community newspapers, shopper's guides, or penny saver magazines. Because these circulations reach a large number of families, and the ads are inexpensive, they are often more cost-effective than placement of ads in the large major dailies (e.g., *New York Times, Washington Post*). Editors of these smaller publications are also more likely to be looking for insertions so that publication "turn-around time" may be quicker. A number of groups have been fortunate in having entire articles written about their efforts in the smaller publications because of the closer ties of such publications to ongoing community events and developments.

Low cost ads for emerging self-help groups can be illustrated by three hypothetical examples.

Example 1:

Need support, encouragement, and people who understand. Join (name of group). Call (person), (telephone #).

This first ad does not indicate a meeting place. It is particularly useful for a group that either does not have a meeting place as yet, is varying its meeting location, or is actively meeting at someone's home and that person does not wish to have his or her address indicated in the ad. Usually the contact person is listed only by first name. This provides a sense of anonymity and security.

Example 2:

(Name of group) now meeting. Call (person), (telephone number).

This particular type of ad can draw members only if the name of the group is specific and distinguishable. Names such as Families of the Mentally Ill, Unemployment Self-Help Group, or Widows Support Group clearly demonstrate the types of persons sought for membership. This ad is slightly cheaper than that illustrated in Example 1.

Example 3:

(Name of group) invites you to attend its weekly meeting: (day), (time), (place).

In this illustration the group is featuring an established place and time, rather than contact person and telephone number. It is important that the location be stable, lest potential members subsequently come to a designation that is no longer in effect.

Whether founders seek publicity in smaller or larger publications, there is a major newspaper fact they share in common. Editors and reporters do not take offense when interested parties call them multiple times about the appearance of a given story. Indeed, it is often assumed that unless there are follow-up calls concerning a delayed story, it is not worth printing. Thus if a newspaper or magazine promises to run the story in two weeks and it does not do so, it would be in the best interest of the self-help founders to call the relevant editor or reporter to determine the current status of the story and strongly urge its appearance by citing the relevant benefits to be derived. A second follow-up phone call should be made approximately 10 days to 2 weeks later to ensure that the story is getting its due on the queue line.

In addition to newspapers and magazines, self-help founders might spend some time trying to determine what radio programs or TV broadcasts are partial toward their cause. Contact with the relevant producers of a show oriented toward community development, health issues, self-care, or social problems would be the most likely types to contact.

Needless to say, publicity via the written or spoken word can lead to receipt of many telephone calls and letters regarding group membership and curiosity about the function of the organization. Founders may again find themselves in the situation with multiple requests exceeding the group's desired size. Thus a careful action strategy should be developed.

The First Meeting

ANNOUNCING THE MEETING

Once the founder (or cofounders) have concluded that there are sufficient numbers for initiating the group, a letter or call should be made to the individuals expressing group interest. Although the former is cheaper and can take less time, a telephone call is much more desirable. Direct conversation enhances the rapport-building necessary for sustained membership; it allows for questioning about the group's purposes, goals, and objectives; it demonstrates a personal concern about the potential member; and it ensures that when the new person enters the group he or she already knows someone—"I am not a total stranger, there is someone I can already identify with."

The first meeting usually begins with the founder welcoming everyone to the group; providing some background information about why there was an attempt to initiate the group; the types of people sought for membership; and the reasons for such selection. These remarks help to put everyone on the same footing; all can now feel as if they have some familiarity with the way *their* group has emerged.

The next and most critical stage is to initiate the rapport-building process. Unless members can develop an effective bonding, there is increased probability that the group (or at least, some subset) will dissolve. This process ordinarily begins with the founder indicating that everyone present shares at least some common experiences, problems, or concerns. Otherwise, they wouldn't have come to a group meeting of this type. "And what better way to learn of what we all have in common than by going around the room, talking about why we've come to this meeting and what we hope to get out of the group."

Discussion of this sort sometimes takes off rather sputteringly. One or two people might be willing to talk outright; others prefer to sit back and see how things develop; still others might be shy; and still others might be cautious about revealing their very deep concerns or feelings.

To help break the ice the founder will often begin, or follow shortly thereafter a more desirous speaker. What must be kept in mind is that no one person be allowed to dominate the group, particularly at a time when it is first developing. Otherwise, potential members may drop out or divide into cliques against such dominant parties. As there is no recognized leadership yet, the founder traditionally plays the role of peacemaker, facilitator, and moderator, trying tactfully to maintain a positive group process.

A situation may arise, however, in which one or more speakers needs to speak more than the fair allotted amount of time. This will occur in those situations where there is a strong need to vent feelings of frustration, anxiety, concern, or guilt. For many individuals, lack of previous access to a support group has resulted in a lot of "bottled up" feelings that need to come out. Group members are often likely to allow such persons the extra time if they, in fact, really require the group's immediate attention. Indeed, the fact that a person can receive at least a modicum of relief in the first meeting helps to bind the group together all the more quickly; they can see that the group really does work.

The initial meeting continues within the preset allocated time frame, providing as many people as possible the opportunity to talk about why they came to the group and what their hopes and aspirations are. As speakers complete their remarks, the founder should demonstrate how closely one's needs and expectations tie to other members of the group who have already spoken. This helps to demonstrate to members that there is a reason to be together, that they have experienced the same emotions and feelings, that they can turn to each other for understanding, empathy, and support. A sense of "belonging" begins to emerge, and with it a group commonality. Given an honest interchange between members, even the first meeting can do much to foster the necessary rapport-building for positive group interaction and development.

Another important aspect that must take place at the first meeting is the planning of the second meeting. When should it be held? Where should it be located? Should efforts be made to contact persons who promised to be at the initial meeting but did not attend? Should everyone pitch in for coffee and cake? For each group this is an individual decision-making process. In general, however, it proves most satisfactory to maintain one standard meeting place; the group's "home," if you will. Ideally that place should be centrally located, in easy transportation reach for the majority of the members. As most groups tend to meet once a week or once every two weeks in the early stages of group formation, the meeting place should be available during those times.

The calling of absentee members is desirable because lack of attendance does not necessarily mean lack of interest. Family or transportation issues, schedule conflicts, or other unforseen events may have prohibited potential members from attending that first meeting.

The Second Meeting

The general tone of the second meeting is very similar to that of the first. Members who did not receive a chance to speak about their reasons for joining the group at the first meeting should certainly be given their due time at this second gathering. For groups with large memberships, almost an entire second meeting may have to be dedicated to member dialogues about why they joined the group and what they hope to obtain from group participation. Although this procedure might seem terminally long to an outsider, group members are often "hungry" to find other people going through the same situations they are confronting, and are oftentimes surprised to find that they are not alone or unique in their feelings. Many anecdotes can be provided detailing the surprised disbelief shared by members hearing others tell a tale similar to their own. The feeling of not being alone, of not being the only one having particular concerns and problems, is reward enough for most people attending the group's first two meetings.

By the second half of the second meeting the foundation of a group spirit should have emerged. It is within this framework that the founder should now broach the issue of the group's direction: What shall be the goals and objectives of the group? Who shall lead the group? and so on.

GOALS AND OBJECTIVES

Although general goals and objectives were casually discussed in one-to-one conversations between founder and each potential members before joining the group, the group need not adhere to those earlier conversations with the individual founding member. That individual now represents only one person out of a larger universe. This point is important for founders and members to understand clearly. There is no necessary subversion of the founder's principles or grounds for initiative; rather, when a multiple number of persons join together, there is bound to be some degree of change; the majority will always have at least some differences of opinion from the founding member.

One methodology the group may use to discuss future goals and objectives is to list suggestions on a blackboard or large piece of paper. After all suggestions have been made, and followed up with the necessary levels of specificity, the group can vote, either by closed or open ballot, on priority ratings. The goals and objectives receiving the highest priority rating scores will receive the major focus of the group. As needs and desires change, new goals and objectives can be formulated. This technique is known as the "nominal group" approach.

In some groups, however, there is less member flexibility. Some nationally based organizations have developed specific formats and/or specific sets of goals that must be followed as a condition of membership. While some creativity is endorsed, members are not free to run their meetings entirely as they wish, nor can they alter the guiding principles or bylaws upon which such groups are based.

It should be indicated that the presentation provided in this chapter is particularly oriented toward those individuals starting a self-help group from scratch, with no encumbrances by any specific formal organization or self-help national/regional office. Obviously in the cases where a new group is getting started as a chapter of a larger organization or group, founders and members must decide if they wish to be guided by preestablished policies, formats, and agendas.

Preestablishment of guidelines should not, of course, be viewed as necessarily detrimental to effective solution or remediation of a given person's problems or concerns. Indeed, in many instances, groups that have developed a preestablished way of doing things have come to adopt these forms because they have been shown to be most workable over time. A new group will sometimes falter until it comes upon the most effective types of group process.

It is, therefore, recommended that for a new group starting out on its own, a subcommittee be formed to visit other more established groups, sit in on their meetings, meet their officers, and see how they handle their affairs. Alternative developmental methodologies can then be discussed, with the pros and cons of each being highlighted.

GROUP LEADERSHIP

Depending upon the progress of group development, another major issue may get raised at the second group meeting. This relates to the role of the founder vis-à-vis other group members. As indicated above, the founder has been playing facilitator, mediator, and arbitrator roles within the group. The question now needs to be raised: Should the founder continue in such capacity as the group coalesces as an entity? Or should the group elect officers, have members take turns leading the group, or exist without formal leadership? By the founder raising such issues, that individual is demonstrating to the group that there is an acknowledgement of a peer-oriented, egalitarian-focused group. No doubt such action will be appreciated by the membership.

Although discussion of this topic may be given some time during the second meeting, it may be conceived more as "food for thought" by members rather than something that needs to be dealt with immediately. Chances are the group will be satisfied with the actions of the founder if all is going well and will probably allow that person to continue in a facilitation capacity until after the more pressing needs of group purpose, aims, objectives, and immediate activities have been effectively managed.

Subsequent Group Meetings

This chapter has been principally oriented toward initiation of the group. As such, focus has centered on membership development and the first two meetings. However, at least the subsequent five meetings are very important as well. It is during those times that the group determines whether members can build and maintain a solid working relationship with one another and whether they can effectively assist each other in meeting their mutual needs.

SIGNS OF POSITIVE GROUP PROCESS

Over time members should be demonstrating a greater capacity to share and "open up" with one another. They should be expressing a willingness to listen to one another, as well as discussing the problems and concerns common to all. For the group to endure, members should be exchanging experiences and providing support, empathy, and encouragement. If this is not happening, a frank discussion needs to be initiated to determine the obstacles or roadblocks to effective group process. Otherwise, a sizable dropout rate is likely to occur.

To maintain a positive working atmosphere, members must also be willing to share tasks and responsibilities and take an active role in dealing with the business issues of the group. It is these common principles that have led support groups to be called "*mutual* aid groups." "Self-help" is, thereby, somewhat of a misnomer. One does not join a support group and find that concentration is focused solely on the individual self. Rather, by all group members helping each other, all gain in the process.

It should be noted, however, that there are certain very shy individuals who take a long time to be acclimated. The group should not push such individuals to assume tasks and responsibilities that the person is not yet ready to take on. One of the hallmarks of a self-help group is that it is not time-oriented. Some people move along at a faster pace than others. As long as an individual is not thwarting the group process, and appears to be trying, necessary time for development should be allocated to that individual.

ISSUES

It is particularly during these subsequent meetings that business issues will concern (a) further clarification of the goals and objectives; (b) specific activities of focus; (c) setting agendas; (d) deciding whether to take on new members and how to deal with dropouts; (e) dues, contributions, and donations; (f) group process as inner-directed versus outer-directed; (g) officers; and (h) relationship to outside organizations.

Talking with other self-help groups of a similar nature, coupled with close attention to membership suggestions and recommendations, should help to ensure that the group's current objectives are meeting the needs of the members. As necessary, discussions regarding change should be placed on the agenda. It should be recognized that change in itself is not good or bad, just a requirement to manage a new situation better.

Agenda setting and focus on specific activities follow from a clear determination of the group's aims and objectives. As in other group process decision-making stages, members should propose what they deem to be in the best interest of the group and of themselves, clarifying the advantages and disadvantages, time lines, costs, manpower, and feasibility. Appropriate voting procedures adopted by the group should then be utilized in the decision-making process. Usually a majority suffices for an activity to be adopted.

How many new members should be sought/allowed to join the group ultimately depends upon the satisfaction of members with their current count. Is there not enough stimulation? Are members too similar or different? Are new recommendations or insights needed for coping or dealing with member problems, concerns, or issues? Is there a desire to help as many people as possible in need? Are more members necessary to perform the desired group goals? and so on. In the case where the group is unsure as to how many more members can be tolerated at a given time, conservatism is probably best.

Trying to ascertain why early members dropped out can be an important task of the group. If the group can come to understand its weaknesses or contributions to dropout, and take the necessary modification steps, further dropout may be either eliminated or diminished. Phone calls to those no longer in attendance would encompass the most personal touch available. Demonstration of group concern may even entice dropouts to return, if appropriate modifications are to be made. Alternatively, a letter may be sent; but there is little reason to believe that the return rate among discouraged members is going to be high.

In terms of dues and contributions, most groups are either free or charge very minimal rates (infrequently more than $10/year). For those unable to pay, either because of a low income scale, unemployment, or other financial necessities, most self-help groups that charge utilize a progressive scale or waive the fees altogether. The hallmark of a self-help group is concern and encouragement of others. Financial capacity is not a primary consideration.

The direction the group takes depends upon membership decisions about the goals and objectives of the organization. Given a continuum, using "inner-directedness" (application of practices toward benefit of its own members) as one point and "outer-directedness" (practices oriented toward those *outside* the membership) as the opposite point, self-help groups must choose their orientation to the universe. Some groups prefer to be inner-directed, concentrating all energies on helping their own members. Other groups are outer-directed, acting in an advocacy capacity to help bring about change, thereby helping themselves in the process. And still others fluctuate between adopting both positions. There is no right or wrong answer. It is simply a matter of choice and need.

With reference to officers, it was indicated above that some groups adopt a stable, continuous leadership with built-in rules for succession; others have a revolving form of leadership, giving each individual a chance to facilitate or lead the group. Still others do not see the need to have officers at all; rather, they just view different members as performing the multiple tasks associated with the group's management and viability. Whichever form is adopted should suit the group's temperament.

The final issue cited concerns the group's relationships to other organizations. This will be taken up separately in the next section, specifically related to the professional community.

Relationships to Professionals

In working with other organizations of a more formal nature (e.g., hospitals, schools, community mental health centers, day-care facilities, churches), self-help groups commonly come in

TABLE 6.3   Positive Professional Staff Impact

(1)   Assistance in group development and facilitation
(2)   Recruitment of initial and subsequent members
(3)   Adaptation and placement of media advertisements
(4)   Provision of a permanent meeting place
(5)   In-depth consultation
(6)   Service on self-help boards
(7)   Self-help group referrals
(8)   Participation on the group's Speaker's Bureau
(9)   Fund-raiser
(10) Colleague on grants/contracts

TABLE 6.4   Negative Professional Staff Impact

(1)   Inability of some professionals to maintain their prescribed role as consultant or advisor; control can become an issue
(2)   In helping to facilitate a self-help group, professionals may adopt a hierarchical, clinical model rather than a peer egalitarian modality
(3)   In monetary relationships of a grant or contractual relationship, principal organizations, departments, services, and individuals must have their obligations and responsibilities agreed upon, lest competition, nonparticipation, and/or control be sought
(4)   Professional board members must be acquainted with the philosophy, goals and objectives, and history of the self-help movement so as to mitigate against selection of noncommunity-oriented personnel
(5)   Credits, acknowledgements, and collaborations need to be carefully worked out so that media publicity is satisfactory to all concerned
(6)   Professional speaker bureaus must be informed of the highly sensitive references and terminologies that can splinter or damage the self-help group's network-building relationships
(7)   The legalities and charges related to utilization of a professional organization's meeting rooms needs to be determined to minimize liability and budget concerns

contact with professional personnel. Although such persons have a lot to offer the support group, a number of conflicts can also be created.

Considering the positives first, professional personnel have the education, training, and experience to assist self-help groups in a multiple number of ways (see Table 6.3).

On the other hand, if not carefully discussed and clarified beforehand, certain damaging relationships may evolve between the self-help group and professional (see Table 6.4).

With these caveats in mind, many self-help groups have worked quite well on a collaborative basis with professional organizations and consultants. Other groups have found it in their best interest to work only with the lay public or their own membership. Again, the choice remains for each particular group to clarify uniquely.

References

Antonovsky, A. (1979). *Health, stress and coping.* San Francisco: Jossey-Bass.

Bandura, A. (1985). Model of causality in social learning theory. In M. J. Mahoney & D. Freeman (Eds.), *Cognition and psycotherapy* (pp. 82-99). New York: Plenum Press.

Berkman, L., & Syme, L. (1979). Social networks, host resistance and mortality. *American Journal of Epidemiology, 109,* 186-204.

Bryant, N. (1983). Self-help and perinatal health. *High Hopes, 3.* Memphis: National Association of Perinatal Social Workers.

Butler, R., Gertman, J., Oberlander, D., & Schindler, L. (1979/1980). Self-care, self-help and the elderly. *International Journal of Aging & Human Development, 10*(1), 95-119.

Caplan, R. (1979). Social support, person-environment fit and coping. In L. Ferman & J. Gordus (Eds.), *Mental health and the economy.* Kalamazoo, MI: Upjohn.

Cassel, J. (1976). The social environment as a factor in host resistance. *American Journal of Epidemiology, 104* (2), 107-123.

Colombotos, C. (1976). In *Preventive Medicine, USA* (p. 37). New York: Forgarty International Center and American College of Preventive Medicine.

Coombs, R., & Fawzy, F. (1985). Adolescent drug use: Patterns and problems of users and abstainers. In B. Forest (Ed.), *Alcohol and drug use in special populations.* Monterey, CA: Wadsworth.

Costello, R. (1976, September/October). Teen age rap groups. *Social Policy, 7,* 2.

Creer, T. (1978). Asthma: Psychologic aspects and management. In E. Middleton, C. Reed, & E. Ellis (Eds.), *Allergy principles and practices.* St. Louis, MO: C. Mosby.

Gore, S. (1978, June). The effect of social support in moderating the health consequences of unemployment. *Journal of Health & Social Behavior, 19,* 157-165.

Harveston, D., Kirshbaum, H., & Katz, A. (1976). Independent living for the disabled. *Social Policy, 7,* 2.

Hayden, A., & Haring, N. (1976). Early intervention for high risk infants and young children: Programs for Down's Syndrome children. In T. Tjossem (Ed.), *Intervention strategies for high risk infants and young children* (pp. 573-608). Baltimore, MD: University Park Press.

Human Services Center Stress Counseling Program. (1983, December 30). *Annual report.* Los Angeles: The Suicide Prevention Center of Los Angeles. (mimeo)

Jones, P. (1982). *Living with hemophilia.* Philadelphia: F. A. Davis.

Katz, A. H. (1961). *Parents of the handicapped.* Springfield, IL: Charles C Thomas.

Katz, A. H., & Bender, E. (1976). *The strength in us: Self-help groups in the modern world.* New York: New Viewpoints.

Lipson, J. (1982). Effects of a support group on the emotional impact of caeserean childbirth. *Prevention in Human Services, 3,* (17), 17-20.

Minde, K., Shosenberg, N., & Marton, P. (1975). *Self-help groups in a premature nursery—a controlled evaluation.* Presented at the National Conference on Social Welfare.

President's Commission on Mental Health. (1978). Vol. II; appendix. Washington, DC: Government Printing Office.

Robinson, D., & Henry, S. (1978). *Self-help and health.* London: Martin Robertson.

U.S. Department of Health and Human Services (1982). *Proceedings, Conference on Alcohol, Drug Abuse, and Mental Health Promotion/Prevention at the Worksite.* Washington, DC: Author.

Van Harberden, P., & Lafaille, R. (1978). *Zelf-hulp.* Gravenhage: Vuga.

White House Report (1977). Conference on Handicapped Individuals Vol. 1. Washington, DC: Government Printing Office.

Chapter 7

MIGHTY OAKS
The Potential of Prevention in the Workplace

SHEILA H. AKABAS

This chapter is about the protection and promotion of mental health in the workplace. Historically, the workplace has not been perceived as a nurturing environment, but rather as a place of drudgery, unhealthful competition, and Darwinian survival, or, more recently, of toxic hazards. This chapter, then, asks the reader to turn a new leaf—to regard what is positive or potentially so about work and the workplace as a source and resource for the protection and promotion of mental health. It will begin with an overview of present day work settings and a rationale for their interest in mental health. The range and characteristics of mental health efforts will be described, as will some of the issues that surround these programs.

The chapter will include a look into the future because the unrealized potential in this arena is greater than present practice and past experience. Sufficient evidence exists to support the assumed relationship between personal well-being, worker satis-

Author's Note: Preparation of this chapter was supported in part by Grant No. 5-T24-MH-14462, ''Systems Approach to Workers and Their Mental Health.''

faction, and productivity so that resources devoted to promoting mental health at the workplace hold promise of cost-effective outcomes. The verification of that reality, however, awaits evaluative research, still undone.

A preliminary word seems in order. The world of work has not invited the mental health professional to enter. Rather, there is ambivalence, and even suspicion on the part of both management and labor toward mental health professionals. In part this can be attributed to fear of the unknown. Mental health professionals, therefore, need to stress their similarities with the work world representives rather than draw attention to their differences. This means something as minor as adopting the dress code of that world, and something as major as becoming informed of its language and demonstrating concern for its single-minded verbal attention to the "bottom line." Many years of experience tell me that once trust is established, however, focus on the bottom line recedes as management and labor take pleasure in being the same kind of do-gooders that they pejoratively accuse mental health professionals of being.

Professionals, whether in-house employees or contractors, need to understand the rationale that can appeal to corporate representatives or union officials concerning the values of prevention mental health services. The wide range of motivations (Akabas, 1984c) runs the gamut from concern about public image to actually wanting to do good, from seeking to attract a better recruitment pool to wanting to respond to community demands for affirmative action. Management, perhaps most important, wants to keep up with the competition. Any argument that correlates profitability with mental health promotion will be welcomed. Unions, too, have a variety of motives, but membership loyalty is their bottom line. Long ago C. Wright Mills (1948) recognized that one of a labor leader's functions is to "organize discontent and sit on it." If service availability will help maintain union loyalty, services are likely to be well received. In short, the professional seeking entry to the world of work to develop mental health prevention and promotion efforts will do well to remember Adam Smith's injunction that self-interest explains most of the world's actions.

THE MEANING OF WORK

As background for the discussion that follows, the meaning of work, the nature of the workplace, and the historic relationship of mental health professionals all seem relevant. Work as an activity has had a checkered reputation starting with Adam and Eve's banishment from Paradise and condemnation to toil for having disobeyed the divine edict. The ancient Romans and Greeks avoided work, believing it to be the effort appropriate to slaves. Renaissance recognition of the opportunities for creativity involved in work, however, was reinforced by the Protestant Ethic's link of work on earth to favorable rewards after death, assuring considerable devotion to work in the Western world. Freud confirmed this view by identifying the ability to love and to work as the hallmarks of adult functioning. Various observers have viewed work as the source of financial support, as an organizing activity that establishes the routine for our life, as an ego-satisfying foundation for self-image, as the definition of our social status in the community, as a social support system through which we derive contacts and friends, and ultimately as a place of opportunity for creativity and self-realization. The work we do tends to determine where we live, how, with whom, the education our children receive, and even their future occupations.

Each of these formulations provides entry points for mental health promotion. For example, if work establishes the routine for our life, then assuring that those who retire gain a positive substitute routine helps provide continued meaning to our existence. If it influences our self-image, then it is preventive to develop a meaningful work experience for teenagers and other age cohorts. Other programmatic interpretations will certainly occur to the reader. Support for such activities may be available from concerned worksites, from community organizations, and from other funding resources that might welcome connection to such a mainstream concept as work. Although we might decry the societal attitude that considers work more important than some other values, we should certainly not overlook those with such attitudes who might be a source of funding for preventive mental health efforts. Although some research suggests that there is a diminishing interest in work, the long lines of job applicants when a new workplace or apprenticeship opportunity opens, or when a civil service test is scheduled, defy the popular wisdom that the work ethic is in decline. There are poignant testimonials about the importance of work. Maurer (1981) quotes a person, fired, as comparing the loss of a job to rape:

> I was persuaded that I must be not only as bad as the company must have thought I was to fire me, but much worse than that. Probably the world's worst. Probably I didn't deserve to live. . . . It's the brutality [of being fired]. It may be more like rape than death.

Feldman (1980) records the comments of another fired victim, a cancer patient:

> I died twice—once when I heard the diagnosis and a second time when my boss heard it, and fired me because of it.

Surely if work can evoke such powerful emotions it must be an important ingredient in mental health.

Work is the focal activity of an American labor force of 114,000,000 persons, a force that increases at a rate of about 2 million persons a year. As is widely identified, that labor force includes increasing proportions of women and minority group members. Yet jobs remain highly segregated, with women occupying two-thirds of all clerical, sales, and service positions, and minority workers disproportionately among the lower-skilled occupations and the unemployed. Such occupational allocation does not promote positive mental health.

Unemployment, although not at a peak, is high, numbering approximately 9 million in 1984. The negative mental health impact of wanting to work and not being able to find employment has been confirmed (Brenner, 1973). Activities directed toward easing job transition and career change would find acceptance among workers and labor unions.

Professionals interested in mental health promotion in the workplace should not overlook the value of advocacy and political action. Legislative and regulatory initiatives have produced many positive gains. Child labor is barred, minimum wages and maximum hours are set, the right to bargain collectively is assured, civil rights and health in the workplace are the subject of legal requirements, private pensions are vested and guaranteed, and the welfare system rewards workers through its social security provisions, to cite just a few examples. Each of these represents legislative action that has contributed to establishing a climate conducive to mental health.

The freer we are to choose our own work, the more likely is its positive impact on our mental health (Sennett & Cobb, 1973). Work can tell a great deal about an individual. Clinically, it is possible to gain understanding of a particular client by reviewing his or her work history and present work situation (Strauss, 1951; Vigilanti, 1982). Neff (1968) has suggested that knowing a worker's ability to perform the assigned task of the job, to meet its routine requirements, and to manage interpersonal relationships with peers, subordinates, and supervisors will provide data needed for diagnosis and treatment as effectively as the more traditional early life history. What jobs require in the way of task, routine, and relationships is relevant to help clients select jobs that fit and/or will enhance their coping ability and promote personal growth. Similarly, management must be aware of the same three factors if they are to provide a climate conducive to the mental health of the labor force.

Not all work, obviously, is viewed as positive and reinforcing. Sennett and Cobb suggest, in fact, that for many people work is demeaning and stigmatizing, resulting in "the hidden injury of class." Interviewing workers throughout the country, Terkel (1972) found some who saw the product of their labor as their posterity, their "astonishment," and others who felt like robots or caged beasts. Levi (1979) has been more specific, identifying some work as causing psychological reactions such as fear, depression, and somatic complaints; behavioral reactions such as alcoholism, drug abuse, and even suicide; and physiological reactions such as cardiovascular disease.

Positive job qualities, on the other hand, include demanding tasks that offer learning experiences and decision-making opportunities, in an environment that provides social support and recognition, and that allows the worker to relate work, positively, to the rest of life. Jobs that match authority with responsibility and offer congenial workmates are also viewed positively. Conversely, NIOSH, for example, has confirmed that boredom and lack of control, in comparison with responsibility, lead to low self-esteem and stress-related diseases (McLean, 1979).

Given the importance of work in people's lives, I believe professionals would contribute greatly to promoting mental health if they improved their capacity to help clients analyze their jobs and its consonance or dissonance with their own needs and expectations. There can be little doubt but that some work can protect and promote mental health whereas other work requires modification if it is not to be detrimental to one's well-being. A few fortunate mental health professionals have been hired in recent years as employees at worksites where they have been able to join with management toward development of work teams, quality circles, and other worksite accommodations that help create a climate more conducive to mental health. This certainly represents an arena for future activity, and the organizational development literature is replete with suggestions for how the professional should proceed.

THE WORKPLACE

The workplace can be conceived of as an environment (Moos, 1976), a tertiary developmental institution, following family and school (Eichner & Brecher, 1979) or community (Klein, 1968). Each formulation leads to the same conclusion—the workplace can be a significant system for preventing mental illness and promoting mental health. The strategy such recognition precipitates, however, varies with the conceptual formulation.

Consider the finding, for example, that environments marked by social isolation are destructive. Researchers studying admissions to mental hospitals found that the rate of admission for blacks living in communities where they constituted less than

10% of the population was excessively high. Similar results were found for Italians. For professionals interested in prevention, concern about the environment extends beyond the hygiene of the workplace (that it be clean and quiet). It is not enough that a workplace hire minority group members or women. Their placement within any specific unit in the workplace should be in sufficient numbers so that they do not experience their employment as tokenism. Placing three women on different assembly lines may be detrimental to mental health, whereas placing three women together on one assembly line may provide sufficient support so that they can function with a sense of well-being. In *Men and Women of the Corporation,* Kanter (1977) provides guidelines for a structural analysis of the workplace that can be helpful to professionals who wish to work with management and labor in dealing with critical environmental issues.

Organizing educational and learning experience, on the other hand, will be foremost if the workplace is classified as a developmental institution. Support for training programs, educational benefits, and, most recently, lunchtime or after-work informational sessions (on such topics as stress management, college planning, and care for aged parents) suggests that management views its self-interest as involved with workers' growth and stimulation. This development has proved particularly auspicious for the consultation and education services of community mental health centers, which have been particularly hurt during this era of gross underfunding of prevention programs.

A format of a series of from 2 to 4 sessions, offered during lunch or immediately after work, has been well received by work organizations. In marketing these programs, it is important that the professional call on his or her capacity to listen well. Because workplaces differ, a program should be fashioned to the presenting needs of the particular workplace. It is, therefore, important to carry out a needs assessment, clarify goals, and negotiate the timing and length of training to meet the particular interests of the site rather than to superimpose a prearranged package. Groups at the workplace can also be quite tenuous and delicate given the sharing of confidential information. In carrying out groups at the worksite, it is important that confidentiality among participants be stressed. Also, it is necessary to keep such groups from becoming gripe sessions for the discontents. Contracting at the time of group formation concerning the purpose of the group and its process is significant, as in most other group situations.

Finally, a strategy of providing social supports will be uppermost if the workplace is regarded as a community. This is in keeping with Klein's view of the community as a source of physical and social security, help and support in times of stress, and the fount of a sense of self and self-worth. Mutual aid self-help groups have been organized in the workplace for different groups: those recently divorced middle managers finding it difficult to cope with their new existence; families with severely disabled children struggling to balance their own and their child's needs; women in nontraditional settings who are experiencing scapegoating; and the recently bereaved. Management has proved to be supportive of these arrangements because they recognize that workers perform more effectively when they are coping satisfactorily with their personal needs.

Clearly none of these concepts (workplace as environment, developmental institution, or community), is in contradiction. Each leads, however, to a slightly different focus of attention, and suggests multiple opportunities for prevention efforts. The key to actually installing them in a particular workplace is to assess the beliefs and values of the worksite and develop a program responsive to that cultural system.

There are over 4 million workplaces producing goods and services in the United States. These employers may be profit-making firms, not-for-profit institutions, or governmental agencies. Over 100 trade unions represent the labor force in the 20% of those workplaces that are organized. Few generalizations could be made that are applicable to such a range of workplaces and trade unions. The majority of the large employers, however, appear to accept the evidence linking mental health to productivity and therefore the inevitable conclusion that concern about employees and their environment, and the achievement of corporate success, go hand in hand.

In promoting this consensus, three widely heralded books have been instrumental. William Ouchi's (1981) volume, entitled *Theory Z,* was the first. Published at the same time that productivity declines and product defects were identified as damaging America's industrial preeminence, the author identified that caring about employees and encouraging teamwork were the secret assets of the Japanese system. Collective decision making, backed by lifetime employment, promotes the kind of wholistic relationships that assure implicit control within the work group and fosters greater care and responsibility for product quality and firm success (more so than the typical system of external control mechanisms prevalent in the United States).

The following year, in *Corporate Cultures,* Deal and Kennedy (1982) suggested that every worksite has its own culture and that companies with a strong culture are the most likely to succeed (success being measured by bottom-line results). Among those, the most successful are likely to be workplaces where the culture values the human being and his or her contribution, and makes that belief clear to its employees. Finally, in the much heralded *In Search of Excellence,* Peters and Waterman (1982) examined a large number of companies to identify the qualities that accounted for excellence. They deduced that productivity comes through people. Rather than writing off American industrial might, they concluded that we can compete effectively and noted, "The good news comes from treating people decently and asking them to shine. . . . The excellent companies treat their rank and file as the root source of quality and productivity gain."

To any mental health professional, these declarations have a logic that is consistent with our knowledge of people and their behavior (Akabas & Akabas, 1982). Because they confirm the obvious, it is surprising that it has taken so long for the link to be recognized by the business community. But Taylor and scientific management had moved business onto the wrong track, having convinced management that the most effective use of labor in the production process was to reduce it to the status of an interchangeable part. Indeed, robots look like they can replace many of those interchangeable contributors of Taylor. What is missing is that today's service workers, and even more-so the knowledge workers who predominate among the new job holders, must bring themselves to the job to be effective! Thus we have reached the era of opportunity for those interested in mental health protection and promotion (Akabas 1984c). And yet, the promise is relatively unrealized. It is appropriate to ask whether American management, with its history of hierarchical organization and bureaucratic rule making, can change its stripes even in the face of evidence that it would be well-served to do so. A positive answer may depend on the way in which mental health professionals grasp the opportunity.

The history of relative disassociation between the world of work and mental health service professionals is a curious phenomena. Certainly some early human service workers such as Jane Addams of the settlement house movement and Josephine Shaw Lowell of the charity organization movement (Germain & Hartmann, 1980) sought to improve the working conditions of women, end child labor, support trade unions, strengthen workers' right to organize and strike, and lead consumer boycotts, all activities built on the understanding that the workplace is a vital arm of the quality of community life. Present day counterparts feature several programs funded by the National Institute of Mental Health, including a grant to Columbia University's Industrial Social Welfare Center designed to develop "a system's approach to workers and their mental health"; and efforts by the Institute for Labor and Mental Health in Oakland, California, to develop support groups designed to help workers experiencing stress at the workplace better understand the interrelationship between their work lives and their more personal existence (Lerner, 1980).

Most of the time, however, human service professionals and the workplace have all but ignored each other, and, like ships in the night, have made specific efforts to avoid contact (Weiner, Hyman, Akabas, & Sommer, 1973). Understanding and overcoming the reasons for this detachment is necessary if human

service professionals are to undertake a serious effort at protecting and promoting mental health in the workplace.

The first explanation can be attributed to ideology. Historically, and even today, much work is considered to be dehuman-
izing by mental health professionals who choose to remain
aloof from such settings. Second, many human service personnel consider ability to work as prima facie evidence of an
individual's ability to function. Workers are, by this reasoning,
not a group in need of service, or at least not in as great need
as others. Given limited resources, those deemed more needy
have priority over employed persons. Further, many professionals believe themselves powerless to effect change in the world
of work and so remain separate from that world, the better to
criticize it! (Akabas, 1983)

This kind of luxurious wallowing does not serve our client
populations. A recent editorial in *Corporate Commentary*
(Rosen, 1984) summed up the advantages of the workplace as
a site for prevention programming:

> Pre-existing organizational structures, convenient settings and
> potentially supportive environments set the stage for industrial
> based programs. Large scale communication efforts and
> promotional campaigns at the worksite—such as company news-
> letters, payroll stuffers, and public displays of group achieve-
> ment—can stimulate interest more effectively than community
> based programs. Incentive strategies, management and union
> support, divisional competition and aggressive follow-up can
> motivate employees.

Although Rosen was writing specifically about health promotion,
the positive qualities of the workplace are, in large part, applicable to the mental health field as well.

A HISTORIC REVIEW

With this backdrop in place, it is time to explore the response
of the work system. Enough has been written about prevention
elsewhere in this volume to assume that the reader is familiar

with the dual approaches of enhancing the coping ability of the target group while remediating the conditions that place them at high risk.

The development, and even more so the promise, of primary prevention support services at the workplace has been the outcome of an evolutionary process. The initial impetus for service delivery was modest and limited. Around mid-century, American management began to identify alcoholism as a significant contributory cause of accidents, turnover, absenteeism, tardiness, excessive grievances, and use of health benefits. That, coupled with the emergence of Alcoholics Anonymous to which some high-level managerial employees began to belong, and for which they advocated, convinced many workplaces that an alcoholism treatment program might be cost beneficial.

These early alcoholism programs established certain significant principles:

- health and mental health of workers is a legitimate concern of the employer and union
- job maintenance is preferable to discharge
- participation should be voluntary
- utilization should be confidential
- intake and assessment should be without cost to the worker/ client (Kurzman & Akabas, 1981).

Experience with these efforts established that it was possible to save some employees from discharge, and that this might be cost effective (Erfurt & Foote, 1977). Also verified was the hypothesis that early mental health care could reduce the cost of providing physical health benefits (Akabas & Donovan, 1983; Donovan, 1984; Foote et al., 1978; Jones & Vischi, 1979). Evidence suggests that emotionally distressed employees who do not have coverage for mental health care tend to somaticize their complaints. The doctors whom they consult, unable to find any physical cause for such complaints, often order excessive numbers of costly diagnostic tests and x-rays in their effort to rule out any serious physical illness. Such expensive procedures become unnecessary when a troubled worker, insured for mental health benefits, is able to seek appropriate care.

Yet many of those who came to worksite programs received limited help because they came so late in the alcoholism disease process that serious damage had already occurred. Even once they stopped drinking, their lives were so complicated by their prior behavior that they required the kind of help putting their world in order that was quite beyond the skills of the recovering alcoholics who staffed the programs. The next steps were obvious. Why not try to reach people before they build a costly record of dysfunctional workplace behavior? If this intervention is useful to alcoholics, what about workers with other kinds of problems? Why not offer a professionally staffed service, easily accessible and destigmatized, to meet the needs of workers regardless of problem, and to intervene with those at risk of experiencing problems before they occur? Indeed, why not?

These questions were being raised at the same time that management began responding to its newly acquired awareness that the well-being and productivity of workers are highly correlated. And so, a long-standing barrier to employer involvement in the lives of their employees began to erode. Thus the 1980s are a period of startling evolution. The expectation that the employer should maintain an arms-length relationship with the employees' personal lives and those of their families has been replaced by an expectation that the employment situation should be aware of and responsive to the personal needs of workers and their family members. Evidence of this evolution abounds in recent program developments:

- employer provision of day care has become more widespread as is evidenced in the extensive inventory provided in a recent book, *Employer-Supported Child Care: Investing in Human Resources* (Burud, Aschbacher, & McCroskey, 1984);
- employees have gained the right to select benefits from a "cafeteria" of benefit packages that are responsive to the varied needs of individual families;
- flextime work scheduling has been established to meet family requirements, as detailed in such excellent guides as *The Job Sharing Handbook* by Olmsted and Smith (1983).

Each of these trends has been the subject of strong advocacy by community mental health professionals who often have been employed, subsequently, to establish such programs in work settings. Consistently, those managers who provide these varied benefits have testified that their availability contributes to employee morale and is reflected in the "bottom line." Specific objective evidence of this accomplishment is all but nonexistent at present.

The almost universal development of employee counseling services at the workplace is another example of this evolutionary trend. They are of particular importance because they serve as an umbrella for many prevention developments. These services, often called Employee Assistance Programs (EAPs), offer confidential, free, easily accessible care to employees and sometimes family members. Because most are the outgrowth of the alcohol prevention movement described earlier, the programs also accept supervisory referrals. Supervisors are trained to identify workers whose performance is not acceptable, and/or who show signs of deterioration. Such persons are referred to the employee counselor for assessment.

No universal model has been developed for these programs. They run the gamut from in-house services to those contracted with outside profit-making firms, local hospitals, family service agencies, or community mental health centers. Most programs are professionally staffed, although a recovering person is often included in the staffing of a large program. Where there is a union, a steward or some other elected or appointed official is sometimes given release time to participate as a staff member as well. At a minimum, these programs offer assessment and referral. Increasingly, they make available a range of social and mental health services that include not only direct counseling of troubled individuals but also individual and organizational consultation on interpersonal dynamics and educational/informational programs described earlier. Each is based on a realization that although *workers* are recruited, *human beings* come to work.

It is understood that these human beings bring with them their own past experience, personal expectations, and family situations. This "human baggage" has both positive/supportive aspects and negative dimensions. The latter manifest themselves in on- and off-the-job problems involving productivity, sick leave, absenteeism and tardiness, and their own and their family members' utilization of health and other benefits. All these represent cost factors to the employer, and to the union if the workplace is covered by a collective bargaining agreement. Further, the community's view of a particular employer, and hence the employer's ability, at a given wage level, to recruit employees best equipped to perform its job, may be affected by the reputation it gains from being attentive to employees and their needs.

Some employers claim that they can document the cost effectiveness of these strategies in the recruitment and maintenance of an efficient labor force (Lanier, 1981). Using such measures as pre- and postrates of absenteeism, tardiness, accidents, benefit claims, grievances, product rejects, and even premature deaths, programs have evaluated their counseling efforts as being cost effective. Recent interest has focused particularly on the ability of investment in employee counseling to containment of medical costs. Although evidence remains spotty, particularly because of the sparsity of evaluation activity, the concept is appealing and represents another avenue being pursued by mental health professionals. With that, it is appropriate now to turn to some more detailed program examples.

A PORTRAIT OF PRESENT PRACTICE

The literature on prevention is replete with a variety of conceptual frameworks that can be applied to prevention activities within the workplace. For purposes here, the formulation of Munoz (1976) will be utilized. He suggests four areas under which prevention can be viewed:

- those that concern developmental or life-cycle approaches;
- those that deal with functional areas;
- those that examine specific disorders;
- those that respond to specific populations.

Despite the overlapping quality of these concepts, it is possible to apply the framework to examples that specifically focus on each. Programs for preretirees exemplify a life-cycle approach; those that involve occupational safety and health in the workplace meet the definitional requirements for functionalism; stress as a syndrome can be reviewed as a specific disorder; and families can be utilized as an example of efforts that respond to specific populations.

Work with Specific Populations

Proceeding in reverse order, consider family units as a specific population that may be defined by their relationship to the workplace. Gulotta (1981) has described the corporate family as one in which the father's work is a family commitment. Stress resulting from transfers, discrete changes within the work setting, and day-to-day commitments may have powerful repercussions on all members, taxing their coping styles. Rather than adopting palliative therapeutic involvement for individuals, the author recommends "corporate reassessment of personnel policies and practices," noting that "the key to prevention is the corporation itself." Because the importance of top managerial personnel is readily recognized by corporations, firms have been programmatically responsive to suggestions involving these individuals. Some human service professionals have been able to market relocation services for corporate families, helping them think through the meaning of a transfer, and to make appropriate plans for the family members. Other corporations have sought the assistance of mental health professionals in evaluating the appropriateness of various candidates for transfer in relation to their ability to handle the situational changes required. Still other corporations have sought consultation on, and evaluation of, their basic transfer policies. One company, whose policy required that any executive, promoted above a certain level, must have served in at least five different locations at which the firm has facilities, abandoned that position when they were made aware of the negative impact these transfer policies had on families.

A creative professional who understands the problems faced by employees and the needs of the corporation can be quite valuable to both. This influence can be exerted from within the corporation or on a contract basis. Neither paradigm is better than the other, but an in-house position requires a large labor force in need of attention, whereas smaller work groups can be more economically served on a contract basis.

The managerial family is not alone in potentially benefiting from the mental health practitioners' attention. A host of other families are comparably defined by their work connection or work status. They include military families, migrant families, families that own and operate their own small business, single-parent working families, dual career families, and unemployed families. One might even say that a family supported by welfare is defined by work—or the lack of it. The issue of interest here is that the needs of these families for preventive interventions are framed by their work connection.

Some years ago I helped a family service agency respond to the needs of policemen's families in a medium-sized city. Police have an extremely high rate of family disruption and individual substance abuse that warrants preventive interventions on many levels. In the particular situation, the concern was expressed around behavioral problems of adolescent male children. They were responding in self-defeating, macho patterns to peer group challenges to prove that they could not be behaviorally constrained, despite their fathers' positions on the police force. The immediate precipitating event was the death of a youngster during a drunken drag race, egged on by just such a need to "prove himself among peers."

An intervention was designed with the dual goals of improving the adolescent community's respect for the role of police (so that their children would be under less pressure/risk) and improving the intrafamily communication in police families (so that their children would develop better coping styles). It was hoped, as well, that a social support group might be developed among the children. This formulation is in keeping with Klein's view of the functional community of work.

Arrangements were made to have police speak at school assemblies and lead discussion groups at high schools. The mayor's office encouraged lower schools to visit police stations. Careful coaching of police preceded exposure lest they confirm by their presentations the very impressions that were behind the challenges to their offspring. Focused groups led by mental health professionals were convened in police homes. Unfortunately, the effort was never evaluated, but the reported perception of pacticipants was that it was helpful.

Another intergenerational conflict around work that threatened the mental health of parents and children took place among foreign-born garment workers in New York. The children, anxious to assimilate into the community, regarded their mothers' sewing activities in ethnic shops as a source of shame. The immigrant mothers, working long hours under difficult conditions to achieve greater financial security for the family, were miffed and unhappy. They typified the double bind identified by Sennett and Cobb, in which workers labor to improve the family's condition only to find themselves and their work rejected by the children. Having obtained financial security and improved social status, children thereafter looked down on the menial work of their parents.

In consultation with staff social workers, the union organized a Saturday recreation program for families in which a part of the day was devoted to the history of the industry, the Union's struggle for recognition, and the contribution of the industry to the American economy. Parental work roles were dignified in a manner that encouraged new definitions among the young people.

There is also general recognition that there are dilemmas mixing parenting and work and that the problems are further aggrandized for the growing number of single parents. Whether the mother or the father is the single parent, they confront more conflicting pressures and demands than the average parent owing to their dual roles as breadwinner and single status. Parent/worker stress is made more fearsome because of the lack of social policies geared to their special needs. Some workplaces have invited mental health professionals on site to train groups in positive parenting, and have offered space and sometimes even release time for attendees. At the same time, millions of workplaces without such prevention programs would appear to be fertile ground for an approach by the interested mental health provider.

Situations proving most difficult to single parents are poor child-care arrangements, inflexible work hours, unexpected overtime, low level of job satisfaction, illness of a family member, and inaccessibility to children while at work. Employee counselors have learned of these problems as they are repeated consistently by clients requesting assistance. Documenting the needs, and proceeding to draw management's attention to them, has been an effective avenue for achieving new policies. Surprisingly, it seems more difficult to establish the initial commitment of a workplace to provide services to employees than to expand services once the first step has been taken. Advocacy, in coalition with parents, or as a consultant to the management, can help change workplace policies to insulate single parent workers.

Prevention efforts are also appropriate for assisting dual-earner families. There is a prevalent but probably mistaken belief today that dual-earner families have increased in number. Rather, our awareness of them has increased because changes in the organization of work have reduced the number of dual earner-home situations. Family farms and small retail establishments have declined in number, legislation has eliminated "homework" as a production modality, and the development of single individual households has eliminated the vast network of homemakers who earned money by operating their homes as boarding houses (Hunt & Hunt, 1982). Thus what is different about the dual-earner family of today is that the principals have far less control over the location of their work and the allocation of their time than earlier. These developments afford barriers to the primary attention the previously at-home worker was able to devote to family responsibilities. The resulting stress is legendary and often damaging. Job sharing, homework, flextime, leaves of absence, flexible vacation time, and enhanced control over site location have become areas for professional intervention according to an authoritative guide by Olmsted and Smith (1983), cofounders of New Ways to Work.

The contribution of such a systems approach to protection and promotion of mental health seems obvious. Many other examples abound, but a sufficient number have been cited to draw the lessons therefrom. There is a symbiotic relationship between families and workplaces, obvious but not often noted. Whereas families count on the workplace for financial support, medical care coverage, and future job opportunities, the workplace counts on the family to nurture its future workers and to buy its products and pay the taxes needed to support communities. Recently, our awareness that the workplace and its demands may interfere with families and their needs has increased. Many preventive accommodations, therefore, need to be identified so that work and family can coexist. They cannot, as was the myth for so many years, exist in parallel but separate worlds (Kanter, 1977a, 1977b).

Work with Specific Disorders

If the family is a specific population to which the workplace can respond with prevention efforts, stress is a specific disease that offers similar opportunities. Stress might well be considered the disease of the eighties. In one national survey, for example, 82% of the respondents indicated that they "needed less stress in their lives." Instructive is the finding of Holmes and Rahe (1967) that many of the factors that cause stress are work related (e.g., change of job, being fired, promotion).

Concern with stress is based on its association with a series of health problems ranging from depression, substance abuse, and suicide to cancer and heart disease. High-risk target groups have been identified (e.g., the bereaved, the unemployed, the promoted, or transferred) and would serve as a worthwhile focus of mental health prevention activity.

At the same time, there is recognition that some stress is essential for a zestful life, and that the "stress syndrome" is amorphic. Stress is understood to be in the eyes of the beholder—that is, individual reactions vary across given "stressful" situations, and particular individuals may react differently to the same situation under variances of time, environmental factors, or personal circumstances. Research has uncovered the presence of mitigating factors, or buffers, that can influence the response to stress (House, 1981). Although buffers, like stressors, vary in their impact, the worksite context (e.g., how significant the employee perceives his or her work to be) and social support (from persons at the worksite) appear to have major buffering effects. Organizing mutual aid self-help groups (e.g., for first-time workers) has been a prevention effort undertaken at some workplaces, and most particularly under union auspice.

Few would doubt the stressful nature of unemployment or its threat. In fact, Brenner (1973) has been able to establish a direct, though lagged, correlation between unemployment and a host of mental, social, and physical health problems. Figueroa-McDonough (1978) identified kinds of services that could prevent such problems from developing (e.g., concrete help with child care during job search periods, supportive behavior on the part of spouse and friends, job information, help with transportation).

During the recent period of high unemployment in industrial areas, and precipitous plant closings, a number of unions have sought assistance from mental health and other community providers, including welfare department representatives (to certify food stamps) and community college faculty (to help with career counseling and the organization of support services for workers facing impending unemployment). Although such efforts do not necessarily result in increased income to providers, they certainly are responsive to presenting needs in the community and have often been the basis for increased public or foundation funding for mental health services.

In some settings, specific responses have been organized to combat particular stressful situations. The police again provide a good example. Chicago has a long-standing prevention program that has been adopted and modified in many other jurisdictions. There, as a matter of departmental policy, any police officer who discharges his or her gun during duty is required, before returning to the station, to spend several hours in a debriefing session with a mental health counselor. The plan for the session is based on an assumption that the retelling of the event will evoke strong affective responses, allowing the individual to incorporate the experience and prevent serious psychological sequela (including post-traumatic stress syndrome.) The five-stage counseling contact, according to Wagner (1982) includes the following:

- an introduction, during which the program is explained and the employee's cooperation solicited.
- a step-by-step report of the incident to encourage an affective repetition of the experience. (Omissions, illogical statements, difficulty in recall, or changes in affect that might indicate that the police officer is having difficulties with the experience are noted. The counselors are instructed to highlight such cues through discussion.)
- anticipation of symptomatology (e.g., sleeplessness, loss of appetite) as normal, stressful outcome reactions.
- stress management techniques are taught and suggested (e.g., physical exercise, seeking social connections).
- summary is given by the counselor and the door is left open for further contact if needed.

The specific methodology is detailed here because this program has significance for police forces throughout the country and for many other workers who experience trauma at the workplace as well: tellers during bank holdups, airline personnel at crash sites, firefighters and medical personnel caring for disaster victims, teachers attacked in urban schoolrooms. Although only verbal reports are available to confirm the effectiveness of prevention counseling in response to trauma at the workplace, the logic of its potential contribution is appealing, and is supported by references in the literature to employer support for its adoption in other relevant settings (Roy-Brisebois, 1983).

This is clearly not the place for a dissertation on the manifold dimensions of stress. Its significance here is that the workplace has been identified as a major carrier of stress and an equally tangible target for remediation of its ill effects. The carrot of potential savings in health care costs has enticed sufficient interest from decision makers so that considerable resources have been allocated to stress reduction efforts. Most of these have required that remediation be performed by the individual through training in such personal coping responses as meditation, exercise, and biofeedback. There do not appear to be any predictable factors explaining worksite selection of a particular strategy for dealing with stress. At most, what can be said is that a worksite is more likely to adopt *some* program the more its culture values its human resources.

There are, however, systematic approaches possible. A number of writers have described how workers within an organization can carry out an assessment of the need for change to reduce stress, and can organize change efforts in response to that need (Brager & Holloway, 1978; Resnick & Patti, 1980). Their books provide blueprints for the professional who might seek to act as a change agent in a work setting. Only a brief overview and amalgam of their models is possible here. Borrowing heavily from Lewin's force field analysis, these writers suggest that persons of relatively low rank in a setting such as the workplace can initiate change successfully. The stages of action include the following:

- *initial assessment,* during which time not only is the problem analyzed and a goal established, but the decision maker needed to approve the goal and the forces that might support or resist the goal are all identified.
- *preinitiation,* during which the change agent prepares the organization for introduction of the new activity or program. This requires building support within the organization by establishing a network of persons involved in the issue, establishing one's own credibility by proving competence in relation to the issue, and increasing visibility around the issue by magnifying any organizational discontent concerning the

issue or problem. (It is at this time that the change agent decides
whether it is possible to proceed successfully.)

- *initiation,* during which period the change agent moves the
  advocacy effort and the advocates to the center of organizational attention.
- *implementation,* during which the decision maker's commitment is gained and ensured and the change is actually
  instituted.
- *institutionalization,* the final stage at which the change is evaluated, standardized, and linked into the organization's
  structure.

Using this model, efforts have been organized to provide
persons suffering from hypertension with a place to take a quiet
break; increase the authority of workers who experience poor
authority-responsibility fit; and improve supervisory acceptance
of nontraditional workers (e.g., black, female) in particular work
sites. The model is designed for the in-house practitioner who
observes a systemic problem. The outside consultant, on the
other hand, usually has the ear of a top executive. Such a professional is in a position to achieve organizational change by
fiat once the executive is enlisted. Such a consultant, however,
must give particular attention to the implementation and
institutionalization phases.

Although stress and its amelioration is the popular issue of
the 1980s, alcoholism as a specific disorder is probably the most
prevalent, damaging, and long-standing, condition. As well, it
is the condition that initially opened the workplace to mental
health professionals, as was noted earlier, and continues to be
the one that most managers are aware of and for which they
may be counted on to support prevention efforts. In response
to concern over substance abuse at the workplace, educational
programs have promoted primary prevention activity while EAPs
through constructive confrontation have made up secondary
prevention efforts. Even those who support the concept of
alcoholism as a disease, however, agree that some excessive
drinking is situational. Some researchers have identified a culture
of drinking that exists at the workplace, and as a result, efforts

at organizational change have been undertaken to eliminate alcohol from staff dining rooms, corporate parties, and as Christmas presents (Fine, Akabas, & Bellinger, 1983). Whatever the strategy adopted, there is no question but that discussions concerning substance abuse are a guaranteed key to the world of work.

A significant recommendation throughout the literature is that the change agent understand the organization well, identify resistance, and desist when it appears that the goal is not realizable. Given these guidelines, it is possible for mental health professionals to enter the world of work and initiate change to protect and promote the mental health of workers.

WORK WITHIN A FUNCTIONAL AREA

It is sometimes difficult to make the distinction between mental health prevention programs and other prevention efforts in the workplace. One is reminded of Gouldner's (1954) finding that miners live with ongoing discomfort at being below ground, and deal with it by taking days off. When pressures become too great, such as news of an even distant mine accident, they absent themselves from work in large numbers. One could imagine that industrywide improved safety in underground pits would have a direct, positive impact on mental health protection.

For most of those who work above ground, mining presents the convincing but extreme case. But the recent movie *Silkwood,* the tragedy at Bhopal, and court cases surrounding asbestos workers and soldiers exposed to agent orange confirm that there are many other work settings that imperil the physical safety of workers.

Uncertainty about the hazards of one's work environment is a circumstance that imperils the mental health of millions of American workers. Occupational safety and health programs, therefore, represent physical and mental health prevention in the workplace. Protecting workers' physical and mental health by regulating potential hazards and attending to the issues of job-related stress, poor job design, and ergonomic realities received considerable attention during the Carter administration. A professional interested in contributing to this area could help organize joint labor-management groups to consider workplace safety. Such committees are mandated by law, but have considerable difficulty organizing and functioning because the members lack the communication skills that can make for successful problem solving. Interested professionals have been particularly welcomed by labor representatives who often offer Saturday meetings to inform their membership and community professionals on these issues.

Another approach has been for professionals themselves to become intrinsically involved with these issues. General informational campaigns are indicated. The gap in knowledge that would allow for professional detection of workplace hazards is appalling. Professionals who hope to assist in this area must become trained to be aware of hazards and detect their resulting symptoms, must learn to ask questions about what kind of work their clients perform and the conditions surrounding that work. Erratic behavior, for example, and memory loss, may be the result of lead poisoning rather than emotional distress. Right-to-know laws can be used to help workers document and prove cases of lead poisoning and other toxic hazards (Shanker, 1982). In addition, to care for the individual, professionals can adopt advocacy roles, providing legislators with recommendations to exert strong economic pressure in the form of high penalties and fines. Negative publicity can also be aroused against those employers who do not provide safe workplaces. Success of these efforts, however, depends on an informed professional community.

WORK WITH DEVELOPMENTAL OR LIFE-CYCLE APPROACHES

Most persons experience the majority of their life transitions while they are in the workforce. The workplace, therefore, is a uniquely appropriate catchment area for reaching people with preventive mental health programs to ease those transitions. Although attention has been given at the workplace to those experiencing first jobs, undertaking marriage, becoming new parents, and even becoming recently bereaved, the most characteristic program interest has been oriented toward preretirees. Recently, concern for this group has been equaled by interest in buffering the separation experience of long-term workers who are not yet candidates for retirement.

Not unlike the unemployed, the mental health of these two groups is promoted by programs that provide concrete information and assistance in creating new supportive ties. Employers and unions have been very willing to invest resources in such efforts, based on their humanitarian responses and fear of potential lawsuits resulting from charges of discrimination. Although the needs of individuals experiencing retirement differ somewhat from those coping with job severance, members of both these status groupings are often the clients of mental health professionals. For example, retirees might be well served by a structured group-learning experience, with or without spouses and/or other family members, in which they explore feelings and expectations concerning retirement and consider such issues as changes in financial status, health care and living plans, leisure time, and legal, community, and family obligations. The Industrial Social Welfare Center at Columbia University School of Social Work has issued a whole series of guides to developing prevention workshops at the worksite.

The key to gaining workplace support for all these program possibilities, whether directed at target population groups, specific disorders, functional areas, or life-cycle events, is connecting the intervention with cost containment, legal responsibility, competitive labor market condition, reallocation of existing resources, or some other dimension of self-interest of the auspices. Even when that is possible, employers or trade unions may be reluctant to become involved in the personal lives of the workforce, although this concern becomes less prevalent yearly, and may be better explained by their wariness about future expectations (and therefore costs) than their devotion to the rights of privacy. An identification of the resources available for prevention is the obvious next step in developing the case for the workplace as a prevention site.

RESOURCES FOR MENTAL HEALTH PREVENTION
AND PROMOTION IN THE WORKPLACE

The occupational social welfare system is made up of the benefits and services to which an individual and his or her dependents gain entitlement as a result of employment. The most widespread provisions are the fringe benefits that cover vacation and sick pay, pensions, and health care costs. But third party carriers, concerned about what they view as the potential of mental health care costs to be expansive and expensive, have built in limitations (e.g., reimbursement only for the care of certain providers for identified mental disorders that require hospitalization). To restrain even further this "top of the line" type of coverage, policies provide cost sharing, deductibles, ceilings on benefits for hospitalization, maximum number of visits, and reimbursable charges per visit. This financially conservative medical approach encourages the most costly care (hospitalization) from the most costly provider (physicians) often late in the illness process when the need for care is likely to be lengthy.

A countervailing option of easily accessible care from a variety of providers for early intervention to those with problems in living has gathered its adherents, supported by evidence that such mental health utilization is frequently offset by reduced claims for physical health benefits. When care is easily accessible, problems need not fester. A worker does not have to translate concern over an adolescent child into a backache to receive attention; does not have to transform marital difficulties into headaches to be eligible for care; does not have to claim pain in the stomach to gain consideration for tension precipitated by worry over an aging parent. Providing up-front insured coverage for mental health care eliminates the need for people to somaticize their living problems to gain cost-free attention. Research confirms that both the cost of diagnostic testing and of palliative care to dissipate the presenting physical complaints declines when such a prevention benefit is available. Recent insurance riders, therefore, incorporate what might be viewed as primary prevention coverage (e.g., payment for parent education preparation, preretirement counseling and outplacement counseling, that is job search assistance upon discharge).

Mental health providers are appropriately concerned about insurance benefits, including the fringe benefit package, because insurance is often the only or major resource that clients have available to cover the cost of care. Professionals can influence the nature and extent of coverage offered to workers and their dependents by pressing the insurance industry to fashion packages to reflect the advances in mental health protection and promotion:

- to expand coverage to include out-patient care,
- to offer benefits in a way that encourages prevention, for example, provide first dollar and full coverage for an array of problems,
- to eliminate the requirement of a DSM III diagnosis and a physician's assessment for eligibility,
- to cover providers who customarily deal with the interpersonal and intrapsychic problems that people are likely to encounter in the course of daily life and whose intervention goals are more closely related to enhancing coping skills than to long-term treatment of identified behavioral or psychological disorders.

Such benefits would not only enhance early detection, promotion, and prevention activities; they would make it accessible to those with limited financial ability. Further, such benefits would destigmatize utilization by carrying a message that functioning individuals (i.e., workers) are expected to need such assistance from time to time.

Anyone planning a prevention effort at the workplace should clarify what is covered by insurance as an important first step in selling a worksite program. Some of the questions that need to be considered are as follows:

- Which workers are covered? (Many workplaces have different coverage for blue- and white-collar, organized and nonunionized employees.)

- What mental health services are reimbursable?
- Are you, as a provider, reimbursable under the plan(s)?
- Are there any provisions for prevention services?

It may be easier to sell a complete prevention package if the services included are not all add-on costs for the employer or union. If you can point out some services that are already insured, receptivity is likely to increase.

Another funding strategy is possible if you represent a not-for-profit community provider. A prevention effort can be financed out of the workplace's philanthropic contributions if direct payment is not necessary. This path has other advantages as well. Philanthropic gifts can create new services that can be made available not only to the worksite but the general public as well. Thus the worksite can become the creative force for persons in the geographic community as well as to the employees in the funding site.

More significant, perhaps, than the bundle of benefits and services represented by the current occupational social welfare system are the extensive fiscal and personal resources of the world of work that are a back-up to that system and can be enlisted to promote mental health care, particularly if the principal auspices believe that new services will be efficient, cost effective, and utilized by employees. Large-scale employers in the corporate, voluntary not-for-profit, and government sectors have shown increased willingness to allocate new resources to the kinds of primary prevention programs that have been described throughout this chapter. The design of these services in the near future will reflect the creativity and systematic documentation supplied by mental health professions. The dilemma of how to cost out what is prevented will be a major concern, but the opportunities for growth are rich.

For purposes here the important facts are that there is interest and resources available at the workplace, that this interest and resource pool can be expanded by well-documented studies, and that the data and conditions necessary for such studies are relatively available in the worksite. Turning that potential into a reality requires a professional who can explain the potential for "bottom line" impact to the workplace manager.

SOME STRATEGIES FOR INVOLVEMENT

It is not an accident that much of the best documented findings on the value of prevention come out of studies in school systems (Anastas & Reinhurz, 1984). The characteristics of school systems that make such studies possible are similar to those available in the workplace. Consider that any particular workplace is a relatively closed community with an extensive system of "social bookkeeping" that includes longitudinal data on demographic characteristics, health history and related claims, occupational information, performance evaluation and promotional records on individuals, and often comparable data on several sites with specific (and therefore as good as controlled) differences. These circumstances are ideal for experimental efforts in which interventions and/or sites can be varied and their outcomes measured by already collected data on a series of variables hypothesized to be influenced by the intervention, as has been well described by Cohen and McGowan (1983) in their chapter entitled "What Do You Do?: An Inquiry into the Potential of Work-Related Research." The guise of research, therefore, offers one avenue for introducing mental health prevention and promotion into the workplace. There are others, of course.

Any mental health professional, or facilities such as a community mental health center, interested in providing prevention services to the workplace might start by posing and answering a few fundamental questions:

- Why is the provider (you) interested in developing these services?
- What does the provider have to offer?
- Has a specific worksite been targeted?
- Does the provider have contacts at the targeted workplace that can assist with the needs assessment and introductory phases?

- Are there related services or benefits already in existence at the site?
- What are the needs of the specific group for whom services are targeted, and how can the provider meet those needs?
- Is the available time and personnel adequate to meet the needs?
- Can insurance and other fees be collected for services?
- What resources are available within the workplace to support the planned activities?
- Can expected offset savings be described?

Marketing efforts can improve prevention services through the workplace for millions of underserved persons. Private sector resources can be enlisted to support such expansions. But providers, regardless of professional affiliation, will have to be clear about the goals, the process, and the evaluation of the outcome (Akabas & Bellinger, 1983).

SOME CONSIDERATIONS, ISSUES, DILEMMAS

The world of work is a scene of rewards and punishment, no matter how much any particular employer may labor to suggest a different message. Those who do a good job in the way the workplace defines it are rewarded with promotions, raises, and job security. Those not so fortunate may be condemned to dead end positions or severance. It is hard to develop trust, and difficult if not dangerous to identify oneself as weak or in any way limited, in such an environment. Yet trust is the vital ingredient of all mental health efforts.

The workplace is unlike most environments in which mental health professionals operate in that its primary business is usually not people processing. The values and ethics of the professional may be different from those of the workplace manager. Clarity of initial contracting between site and professional and then between professional and client is absolutely essential, as is the ability to protect confidentiality and to act on behalf of clients only under conditions of informed consent (Akabas, 1984a).

Even when these precautions are taken, further contingencies require attentive planning. What happens to the worker who "fails," and develops mental health problems? Or the one who refuses to participate, although referred? As prevention efforts increase, it will be important to assure protection for those who refuse to participate, and services for those who need them, without, "blaming the victim." This is especially important where a person's livelihood is involved.

Employers' self-interest mandates an aggressive policy of showing employees that management cares about them, and about helping them to maintain their maximum well-being. The same is true for trade unions. But like all institutions in our society, there is a great diversity among employers and trade unions—some will be more foresighted than others and, therefore, will behave more forcefully in conveying this message to workers. Because the potential for partnership within the world of work is vast, the mental health provider would do well to invest energy in bringing along those sites where the propensity to act on prevention is evident. Fortunately, such places can often be identified because they exemplify growth in other areas as well. Yet this raises the dilemma of providing prevention programs for those who may need it least. We trust that the synthesis is just around the corner. In the competitive world of work, change has a way of snowballing. Firms tend to jump on the "band wagon" once cost-effective programs have been implemented elsewhere. With hope, but without untoward optimism, it is possible to see the entire world of work as a fertile turf for prevention. The rest is up to the professional community and its ability to negotiate and implement useful "bottom line," quality programs.

References

Akabas, S. H. (1983). Industrial social work: Influencing the system at the workplace. In M. Dinerman (Ed.), *Social work in a turbulent world* (pp. 131-141). Silver Spring, MD: National Association of Social Workers.

Akabas, S. H. (1984a, Summer). Confidentiality: Values and dilemmas. *Social Work Papers, 18,* 83-91.

Akabas, S. H. (1984b, September/October). Workers are parents, too. *Child Welfare, LXIII,* 387-399.

Akabas, S. H. (1984c, December). Expanded view for worksite counseling. *Business and Health, 2,* 24-28.

Akabas, S. H., & Akabas, S. A. (1982, May). Social services at the workplace: New resource for management. *Management Review,* 15-20.

Akabas, S. H., & Bellinger, S. (1983, July/August). Identifying and reaching out to work organizations. *EAP Digest,* pp. 38-48.

Akabas, S. H., & Donovan, R. (1982). *Cost containment and cost benefit analysis in employee counseling programs: An annotated bibliography.* New York: ISWC, Columbia University School of Social Work.

Akabas, S. H., & Krauskopf, M. (1984). *Families and work: Creative workplace responses to employees with disabled children.* New York: ISWC, Columbia University School of Social Work.

Akabas, S. H., & Kurzman, P. (Eds.). (1982). *Work, workers and work organizations.* Englewood Cliffs, NJ: Prentice-Hall.

Anastas, J. & Reinhurz, H. (1984, January). Gender differences in learning and adjustment problems in school: Results of a longitudinal study. *American Journal of Orthopsychiatry, 54,* 110-122.

Brager, G., & Holloway, S. (1978). *Changing human service organizations.* New York, Free Press.

Brenner, H. (1973). *Mental illness and the economy.* Cambridge, MA: Harvard University Press.

Burud, S., Aschbacher, P. & McCroskey, J. (1984). *Employer-supported child care,* Boston: Auburn House.

Cohen, J., & McGowan, B. (1982). What do you do? An inquiry into the potential of work-related research. In S. H. Akabas & P. Kurzman (Eds.), *Work, workers, and work organizations,* (pp. 117-144). Englewood Cliffs, NJ: Prentice-Hall.

Deal, T., & Kennedy, A. (1982). *Corporate cultures.* Reading, MA: Addison-Wesley.

Donovan, R. (1984, Summer). The dollars and 'sense' of human services at the workplace: A review of cost-effectiveness research. *Social Work Papers, 18,* 65-73.

Eichner, A., & Brecher, C. (1979). *Controlling social expenditures: The search for output measures.* Montclair, NJ: Allanheld, Osmun.

Erfurt, J., & Foote, A. (1977). *Occupational employee assistance programs for substance abuse and mental health problems.* Ann Arbor, MI: Institute of Labor and Industrial Relations.

Feldman, F. (1980). *Work and cancer health history: Study of blue collar workers.* Los Angeles: Division of the Cancer Society.

Figueroa-McDonough, J. (1978, September). Mental health among unemployed Detroiters. *Social Service Review, 52,* 383-399.

Fine, M., Akabas, S., & Bellinger, S. (1982, September). Cultures of drinking: A workplace perspective. *Social Work, 27,* 436-440.

Foote, A., et al. (1978). *Cost effectiveness of occupational employee assistance programs.* Ann Arbor, MI: Institute of Labor and Industrial Relations.

Germain, C., & Hartmann, A. (1980, May). People and ideas in the history of social work practice. *Social Casework, 61,* 323-331.

Gouldner, A. (1954). *Patterns of bureaucracy,* New York: Free Press.

Gullotta, T., & Donohue, K. (1981, February). Corporate families: Implications for preventive intervention. *Social Casework, 62,* 109-114.

Holmes, T., & Rahe, R. (1967, August). The social readjustment scale. *Journal of Psychosomatic Research, 11,* 213-218.

House, J. (1981). *Work stress and social support.* Reading, MA: Addison-Wesley.

Hunt, J., & Hunt, L. (1982). Dual-career families: Vanguard of the future or residue of the past? In J. Aldous (Ed.), *Two paychecks* (pp. 41-60). Beverly Hills, CA: Sage.

Jones, K., & Vischi, T. (1979). *Impact of alcohol, drug abuse and mental health treatment on medical care utilization.* Supplement of *Medical Care.* New York: J. B. Lippincott.

Kanter, R. (1977a). *Men and women of the corporation.* New York: Basic Books.

Kanter, R. (1977b). *Work and family in the United States: A critical review and agenda for research and policy.* New York: Russell Sage Foundation.

Klein, D. (1968). *Community dynamics and mental health.* New York: John Wiley.

Kurzman, P., & Akabas, S. (1981, January). Industrial social work as an arena for practice. *Social Work, 26,* 52-60.

Lanier, D. (1981, January/February). Industrial social work: Into the computer age. *EAP Digest,* pp. 18-21, 33.

Lerner, M. (1980). Stress at the workplace: The approach of the Institute For Labor and Mental Health. *Catalyst,* pp. 75-82.

Levi, L. (1979). Psychosocial factors in preventive medicine. *Healthy People: The Surgeon General's report on health promotion and disease prevention background papers 1979.* U.S. Dept. of Health, Education, and Welfare, Public Health Service (DHEW [PHS] Publication No. 79-55071A). Washington, DC: Government Printing Office.

Maurer, H. (1981). *Not working.* New York: New American Library.

McLean, A. (1979). *Work stress.* Reading, MA: Addison-Wesley.

Mills, C. W. (1948). *The new men of power, America's labor leaders.* New York: Harcourt Brace Jovanovich.

Moos, R. (1976). *The human context: Environmental determinants of behavior.* New York: John Wiley.

Munoz, R. (1976). The primary prevention of psychological problems. *Community Mental Health Review, 1,* 1, 5-15.

Neff, W. (1968). *Work and human behavior.* New York: Atherton.

Olmsted, B., & Smith, S. (1983). *The job sharing handbook.* New York: Penguin.

Ouchi, W. (1981). *Theory Z.* Reading, MA: Addison-Wesley.

Peters, T., & Waterman, R. (1982). *In search of excellence: Lessons from America's best run companies.* New York: Harper & Row.

Resnick, H., & Patti, R. (1980). *Change from within.* Philadelphia: Temple University Press.

Rosen, R. (1984, November). From the editor. *Corporate Commentary, 1.*

Roy-Brisebois, M. (1983). Victim assistance: An example of meeting the work-related needs of employees. In R. Thomlison (Ed.), *Perspectives on industrial social work practice* (pp. 123-132). Ottawa: Family Service Canada.

Sennett, R., & Cobb, J. (1973). *The hidden injuries of class.* New York: Vintage.

Shanker, R. (1982, September). Workers at risk: The battle for occupational health. *Practice Digest, 5,* 18-22.

Strauss, E. (1951, November). The caseworker deals with employment problems. *Social Casework, XXXII,* 388-392.

Terkel, S. (1972). *Working*. New York: Pantheon.

Vigilante, F. (1982, May). Use of work in the assessment and intervention process. *Social Casework, 63.*

Wagner, M. (1982). Counseling police officers. *Practice Digest, 5,* 30-31.

Weiner, H., Akabas, S., & Sommer, J. (1973). *Mental health care in the world of work.* New York: Association Press.

Chapter 8

PLANNING PREVENTION PROGRAMS FOR OLDER PERSONS

SHARON SIMSON and LAURA B. WILSON
With the assistance of Stephanie FallCreek, Ray Raschko,
Ruth Loewinsohn, and Nancy Wilson

Older persons are the fastest growing age cohort in the United States. Currently, those 65 and over constitute 12% of the U.S. total population; by 2020 that figure will reach 17% (U.S. Senate, 1982). The health and mental health needs of the older population are great (Butler & Lewis, 1982; Selby & Schechter, 1982). Although the acute and chronic disease problems of the elderly have received much attention, it is only recently that older persons have come to be viewed as a significant target population for disease prevention and health promotion efforts (NRA Planning Panel, 1982; Wilson, Simson, & McCaughey, 1983).

A number of programs are being developed and implemented in various geographical areas of the United States that address the needs of older persons for prevention and promotion activities in health and mental health (Dychtwald, 1983). Many additional programs are needed. One strategy for developing successful programs is to understand the experiences of already established and viable programs. Following the case study approach used in organizational management education, this chapter examines a selection of "best practice" models as a means of assisting others in planning similar programs for the elderly.

HEALTH AND MENTAL HEALTH OF THE ELDERLY

Contrary to some of the myths about aging, most older people lead active, useful lives in the community (Binstock & Shanas, 1976). This day-to-day wellness of older persons is affected adversely by the impact of "lifestyle" diseases (Fallcreek & Mettler, 1982). Despite the significant advances that modern medicine has made in the treatment of acute problems, lifestyle dieseases such as heart disease, cancer, stroke, accidents, mental illness, and diabetes remain a pressing concern (USDHHS, 1980). These diseases are disruptive to the everyday lives of the elderly and are leading causes of death. They are strongly linked to risk factors such as cigarette smoking, poor nutrition, lack of regular exercise, and chronic stress. Approximately 80% of the elderly suffer from one or more of these lifestyle diseases and about half of all older people are restricted in some activities of daily living (USDHEW, 1979).

Although inextricably linked with health, mental health problems are a particular concern because of the high-risk situation of the elderly (Busse & Blazer, 1980). Older persons find themselves having to make major adjustments in later life due to changes in role and status, financial difficulties, new leisure lifestyles, changes in relationships, loss of loved ones, experiences of loneliness and isolation, and alterations in health and physical appearance (Davis, 1983). The Committee on Aging, Group for the Advancement of Psychiatry (1983) reports,

Mental illness is more prevalent among the elderly than among younger adults. Seven studies to date show that 18 to 25 percent of older persons have significant mental health problems; these studies indicate that about 10 percent of older people have neurotic disorders.

The report presents other vital facts about mental health and the elderly. Suicide is more common in the elderly than in any other age group. Psychosis increases significantly after age 65. Senile dementia is considered by some authorities to be the fourth leading cause of death. Many older people experience significant psychological reactions from stress caused by loss of health. Many physical illnesses cause and even present with mental disturbances.

PREVENTION AND PROMOTION
REGARDING THE ELDERLY

Prevention of mental illness and promotion of mental health in the elderly require innovative approaches. In contrast to younger persons for whom prevention efforts are initiated before the expression of the disease, prevention and promotion activities for the elderly tend to be directed at persons who already have one or more chronic disease conditions and may be at-risk of acute illness (Filner & Williams, 1981). Instead of expecting to cure, totally reverse, or completely prevent a disease condition, prevention and promotion programs for the elderly should be directed at altering, modifying, and delaying futher decline (Gaitz & Varner, 1980). The goal should be to increase an elderly person's capacity for improving the quality of life (Kessler & Albee, 1975).

Specific problems of late life may be alleviated or reduced through particular interventions and service delivery systems (Gaitz & Varner, 1980). The design and implementation of programs that address specific diseases or problems such as stress management can reduce an individual's risk of poor health and mental health and provide a starting point for developing more encompassing programs. These prevention and promotion programs attempt to "improve the health and well-being of individuals and communities by providing people with the information, skill, services, and support needed to undertake and maintain positive lifestyle changes" (Fallcreek & Mettler, 1982, p. 2). This approach to prevention and promotion programs for the elderly is in keeping with a holistic perspective, which considers "the human mind, body, and spirit and the social, economic, political, and environmental networks within which the individual lives" (Dychtwald, 1983, p. 2).

BEST PRACTICE MODELS

Individuals and organizations responsible for planning prevention and promotion programs in mental health and/or health for the elderly can benefit from prior efforts made by other programs. Although such programs tend to be relatively new, a number of excellent programs are operating that can provide useful information and insights into the planning process. The following descriptions of selected best practice models represent a range of purposes, approaches, and settings. The models are illustrative of current, state of the art initiatives in aging that include a focus on prevention and promotion as an integral part of an overall health and mental health program. Not all existing programs with such initiatives could be included. Instead, the intent is to provide reviews of several noteworthy programs as an informational base to support future planning efforts.

The four programs reviewed include the following: the American Association of Retired Persons and its Widowed Persons Service; the Spokane Community Mental Health Center Elderly Services; the Texas Research Institute of Mental Sciences and its Texas Project for Elders; and the Wallingford Wellness Project. Program documents and structured interviews were used to collect data about each of these programs in terms of eight topics:

(1) Background: What are the origins of the program? Why was it established? When? By whom?
(2) Objectives: What are the goals, objectives, and purposes of the program?
(3) Programs: What services and activities are offered to clients?
(4) Staff: What types of staff are needed? How many are necessary? What are their tasks?
(5) Clients: What population does this program serve? How many people are affected? What are the characteristics and needs of clients? Are there eligibility requirements?

(6) Organizational relations: What linkages does the program have with other organizations?
(7) Finances: What is the budget for the program? What are the sources of funding?
(8) Contact information: Who can be contacted for additional information about the program?

Information about these eight topics is presented for each of the four best practice models of prevention and promotion programs in health and mental health for the elderly.

BEST PRACTICE MODEL 1: AMERICAN ASSOCIATION OF RETIRED PERSONS AND ITS WIDOWED PERSONS SERVICE

Background

The American Association of Retired Persons is the largest association of retired persons in the world. AARP was founded in 1958 under the leadership of Dr. Ethel Percy Andrus and members of the National Retired Teachers Association. The development of local chapters throughout the United States was facilitated by contacts made by Dr. Andrus and her associates through personal relationships, correspondence, and visits to communities. As of 1984, the AARP had over 3,100 chapters, 13 million members nationwide, and 22,500 volunteers.

The motto of AARP, "To Serve, Not to be Served," conveys the Association's positive and assertive approach to living. The four purposes of AARP reflect factors that contribute to the health and mental health of older persons. These purposes are to do the following: (1) enhance the quality of life for older persons; (2) promote independence, dignity, and purpose for older persons; (3) lead in determining the role and place of older persons in society; and (4) improve the image of aging.

AARP offers educational and service programs that have been designed by and for older people in order to promote "independence, dignity, and purpose" for all older Americans. AARP programs include Consumer Affairs, Criminal Justice,

Driver Improvement, Energy Conservation, Health Advocacy, Intergenerational Activities, Interreligious Liaison, Leadership Development, Lifetime Learning, Program Development, Reminiscence, Safety, Second Career Opportunities, Tax-Aide, and Widowed Persons Service.

It is this last program, Widowed Persons Service (WPS), that serves as a model case and illustration of how AARP programs promote the general health and mental health of its members. Initiated in 1973, WPS was a response to research conducted by Dr. Phyllis Silverman at Harvard that found that widowed persons received the most meaningful recovery help from those who had been through a similar grief experience. AARP is the first organization making a nationwide effort to develop programs to serve the newly widowed.

Objectives

"Widowed Persons Service (WPS) is designed to identify the leadership and resources within a community that will publicly offer services to the newly widowed and help them regain their sense of equilibrium and well-being. The program is based on the concept that significant help can come from someone who has survived a similar experience and is willing to share the trauma of another" (Baldwin & Loewinsohn, 1982).

Programs

In 1984, 142 WPS programs operated throughout the United States. Half of these WPS programs were initiated since 1980, with the first program having been established in 1972. These programs serve as a nucleus of growing networks of helping individuals and community resources for the widowed. Five types of programs are offered through AARP's WPS:

Outreach. The orderly process of contacting, in so far as possible, all newly widowed persons and offering them visits by and communication with widowed people who have adjusted to widowhood and are prepared to discuss openly, on a one-to-one basis, problems that confront the newly widowed.

Telephone Service. A local telephone number is widely publicized to inform the community about the program and enable individuals to request information or service from WPS.

Group Sessions. In response to demonstrated needs of the community and availability of leadership, meetings are held for newly widowed and/or persons who have been widowed longer. These meetings provide a situation in which people with a common bond can discuss issues, learn how to help each other, and initiate social and personal contacts.

Public Education. Through local organizations, public services agencies, workshops, and the media, the program and the needs of widowed persons are brought to the attention of the community.

Referral Service. Each community has organizations and professional personnel to whom widowed persons can turn. Each WPS develops a directory and relationships to provide referral to local services and appropriate agencies or personnel. (Baldwin & Loewinsohn, 1982)

Staff

A local WPS team is made up of volunteers who are willing to give their time and effort to participate in one or more of the services offered by WPS. A typical team comprises about 20 "middle-aged" (51-60) or older volunteers who carry out four main types of roles and responsibilities. The coordinator is responsible for overseeing and coordinating WPS on a daily basis, according to the policies and procedures set by the board. Team leaders are responsible for assignments to volunteer aides, assisting in flow of records, and continuation of aide training. Volunteer aides are responsible for contacting the newly bereaved to offer assistance in coping with and adjusting to the death of a spouse. These volunteer aides have been widowed 18 months or more, have received appropriate training, and have demonstrated recovery from their own grief. The records supervisor keeps track of referrals and obituary information and assignments of aides. This local WPS team is backed up by a national WPS volunteer organizer, a national volunteer trainer, and the WPS at AARP's main offices in Washington, D.C. (Baldwin & Loewinsohn, 1982). In 1984, WPS utilized about 4,000 volunteers in its 142 programs (Prisuta, 1984).

Clients

Widowhood occurs in the United States at an average age of 56. WPS's target population, the newly widowed, are generally defined as having been widowed 45 to 365 days. Although WPS serves many older persons, it was not designed as an "aging" program exclusively but serves widowed persons of any age. WPS programs function in over 170 communities throughout the United States; over 75 additional programs are in various stages of planning (American Association of Retired Persons, PF2136 1082). WPS served approximately 25,000 persons in 1983. The average service area has a population of 340,000; half the programs served 100,000 persons or less (Prisuta, 1984).

Organizational Relations

Widowed Persons Service "supports mutual help programs for the widowed by providing organizational, consultative, recruitment and training assistance, as well as publishing materials available to individual programs and to the public. A cornerstone of the WPS organizing effort is the coalition approach whereby WPS programs bring together the resources of local religious organizations, educational institutions, social service agencies, professional associations, fraternal and service clubs, health and mental health facilities, and AARP groups in a coordinated effort to serve the newly widowed.... Each Widowed Person Service program functions locally under the umbrella of the national WPS" (American Association of Retired Persons, PF1473 980).

The main steps in the WPS organizational process are as follows:

(a) WPS is contacted by a community representative for information;
(b) WPS responds to the inquiry by sending information;

(c) a WPS volunteer organizer assesses the potential for WPS in the community;

(d) a WPS organizer and local representatives work together to hold a community meeting during which a consensus is reached to go ahead or not;

(e) an organizational meeting is held to develop the local WPS program;

(f) training of volunteer aides occurs;

(g) the local program begins;

(h) WPS provides ongoing consultation and support for local WPS program.

Finances

The WPS program is basically operated by volunteers. No fees are charged for services. All operating expenses are kept at a minimum; rent-free offices and borrowed equipment are used whenever possible. In 1984, more than two out of every three programs reported operational support from groups other than AARP. Churches, other aging organizations, health organizations, funeral directors, and community centers were typical supporters (Prisuta, 1984). WPS budgets may run as much as $3,000 per year in contrast to programs with paid personnel that may cost in excess of $100,000 annually. A local program is expected to become self-maintaining.

Contact Information

Contact Ruth J. Loewinsohn, Manager, Social Outreach Services, American Association of Retired Persons, 1909 K Street N.W., Washington, D.C. 20049. (202) 728-4370.

BEST PRACTICE MODEL 2: SPOKANE COMMUNITY MENTAL HEALTH CENTER ELDERLY SERVICES

Background

Elderly Services was established in 1978 by the Spokane Community Mental Health Center. Funding and technical assistance were provided by the Eastern Washington Area Agency on Aging. These agencies had agreed that those elderly who were at-risk for premature or unnecessary institutionalization would be the target group for a network of interdependent mental health and aging services. These services were designed to prevent institutionalization by improving the quality of life of the elderly and maintaining them in their own homes. The program developed by the aging and mental health agencies was influenced by two key considerations: (1) the mental health needs of the elderly cannot be separated from their physical, social, and economic needs, and (2) those high-risk elderly without a support system to act on their behalf tend not to present themselves and their problems to helping agencies and are generally highly resistant to intervention (Raschko, 1984).

Objectives

The activities of Elderly Services have been guided by four interrelated objectives: (1) build a community-based long-term care system in Spokane; (2) prevent premature institutional placement of the elderly; (3) maintain older persons in their own homes; (4) create a core community agency that will take ongoing care responsibility for at-risk elderly living in the community (Raschko, 1984).

Program

Elderly Services offers health and mental health programs with prevention components to clients through multidisciplinary in-home assessment, treatment/service plan, implementation of case management, crisis intervention, supportive counseling, and continuity of care. Elderly Services has used an innovative out-reach method, called the "Gatekeeper Approach," to locate at-risk elderly for referral to its program. In-home case managers for specific geographical areas proactively contact various "gatekeepers"—individuals, agencies, and organizations that are in a position to identify high-risk elderly (Raschko, 1981). Gatekeepers are nontraditional referral sources trained to identify and locate high-risk elderly living in the community who would not self-refer and who do not have relatives or others to act on their behalf.

A valuable component of the community-based long-term care system, gatekeepers include the following: residential property appraisers; apartment managers; postal carriers; meter readers from local electrical, natural gas, and water utilities; fuel oil dealers; the Spokane police, fire, and sheriff's departments; grocery stores; pharmacies; churches; and ambulance companies. Elderly Services conducts regular training programs for these gatekeepers and staff has maintained regular contact with them. During 1983 these gatekeepers accounted for 30% of the referrals to Elder Services. Other referral sources were relatives and friends (22%), other community agencies (19%), physicians and hospitals (16%), area agencies on aging (9%), and self (4%) (Raschko, 1984).

The preventive aspects and method of operation of the Gatekeeper Approach is exemplified by the Postal Alert program. This program is made up of four steps: (1) Elderly persons register for the program at publicized sites; (2) home mailboxes of the elderly are marked so postal carries know which persons are participating; (3) the carrier notifies Elderly Services if mail is not removed from a mailbox; and (4) Elderly Services investigates why mail has not been removed by calling the enrolled person, sending a staff person to the home, and, if necessary, notifying police and taking other appropriate action.

Staff

The staff for in-home case management consists of twelve case managers, one pharmacist/case manager, three field supervisors (two of whom are registered nurses), one part-time psychiatrist, resident physicians, and one program coordinator (Master's in social work). Telephone information and referral is staffed by two full-time telephone screeners (Raschko, 1984).

Clients

Nearly 55,000 persons (16% of the total population) in Spokane County were 60 years of age or older according to the 1980
census. Of the total population, 58% are female and 42% are
male, 2% are members of minority groups, and 32% are 75 years
of age or older. Over 90% lived in their own homes or apart-
ments. Nearly 16% lived at or below the official poverty level.
In 1983, 744 persons were admitted to the Elderly Services
in-home case-management program. Problems presented were
the following: chronic physical illnesses (68%), social isolation/
lack of support system (66%), personal care/activities of daily
living (64%), emotional depression (60%), environmental/social
stress (57%), denial of illness/problems (55%), and memory
impairment (43%). These data are further evidence of the multiple and interrelated nature of the problems experienced by
at-risk elderly. Because of the severity of the problems, Elderly
Services' clients remain active clients for long periods of time
(Raschko, 1981).

Organizational Relations

There have been 14 written coordination and referral agreements negotiated with other agencies, most of which are funded
by the Eastern Washington Area Agency on Aging (Raschko,
1981). These agreements delineate each agency's role, referral
mechanisms, methods of resolving problems, and the sharing
of training and other resources. As a core agency in a network
of biopsychosocial services, Elderly Services is highly dependent
upon other community agencies for the implementation of much
of its treatment/service plan. Among the types of services provided by these agencies are chore services, home health services,
day treatment, minor home repair, telephone reassurance, nutrition and home-delivered meals, hospice, crime prevention, legal
services, transportation, health screening, and newspaper.

Finances

The 1984-1985 annual budget totaled $455,175. The major
contributor, the Eastern Washington Area Agency on Aging,

allocated $267,324 to Elderly Services. This contribution was based on the Older Americans Act ($152,869) and the Washington Senior Citizens Services Act ($114,455). A Washington State grant-in-aid provided $157,851 and the National Institute on Drug Abuse awarded $30,000.

Contact Information

Contact Ray Raschko, M.S.W., Coordinator, Elderly Services, Community Mental Health Center, South 107 Division Street, Spokane, Washington 99202.

BEST PRACTICE MODEL 3:
TEXAS RESEARCH INSTITUTE OF MENTAL SCIENCES
AND ITS TEXAS PROJECT FOR ELDERS

Background

One response to the large and rapidly growing need for long-term care for the functionally impaired elderly is the Channeling Demonstration Program funded in 1981 by the U.S. Department of Health and Human Services. This project is intended to test the feasibility and cost-effectiveness of an alternative community-based long-term care service delivery concept that would integrate health and social service interventions as a means of preventing institutionalization of high-risk elderly. Ten projects in ten different states have been funded to implement the Channeling Program. Project development began in 1981 and sites achieved full caseloads in mid-1983.

One of these channeling demonstration contracts has been administered by a long-time leader in the fields of mental health and aging, the Texas Research Institute of Mental Sciences (TRIMS) Gerontology Center. TRIMS was established by the Texas state legislature in 1958 to provide a complete range of psychiatric services for patients of all ages in Houston and the surrounding metropolitan area of Harris County (N. Wilson et al., 1983). The TRIMS project, the Texas Project for Elders, is the focus of the following discussion.

Objectives

The core objectives of the Texas Project for Elders were identified by the Department of Health and Human Services in its
request for demonstration site proposals from states. These
objectives are as follows:

(1) to marshall and direct long-term care resources in a com-
    munity in ways that contain overall costs;
(2) to increase access to a wider range of services than is currently
    available;
(3) to match services used to the identified needs of the client;
(4) to concentrate public resources on those persons with the
    greatest need for subsidized long-term care;
(5) to stimulate the development of needed in-home and com-
    munity services that do not exist or are in short supply;
(6) to reduce the unnecessary use of publicly subsidized long-
    term care services, including costly medical and institutional
    services;
(7) to promote efficiency and quality in community long-term
    care delivery systems;
(8) to promote a reasonable division of labor among informal
    support systems (including families, neighbors, and friends),
    privately financed services, and publicly financed care; and
(9) to maintain or enhance client outcomes, including physical
    and mental functioning and quality of life.

Programs

Channeling, a relatively new word, describes the specific intervention used in this project to arrange and coordinate the services
needed by impaired individuals in a community setting. Case
management services are provided in cooperation with community agencies to help an impaired person gain access to
coordinated health, mental health, social, and other services as
needed (Gottesman, 1981). Channeling is intended to affect client
outcomes (specifically institutionalization) and the cost of care
by managing individually a client's utilization of service.

The Texas Project for Elders as well as the other channeling projects perform seven essential functions in this channeling process:

(1) Outreach to identify and attract the target population.
(2) Screening to determine whether an applicant is part of the target population.
(3) Comprenehsive needs assessment to determine individual problems, resources, and services needs.
(4) Care planning to specify the types and amounts of care to be provided to meet the identified needs of individuals.
(5) Service arrangement to implement the care plan through both formal and informal providers.
(6) Monitoring to assure that services are provided as planned and modified as necessary.
(7) Reassessement to adjust care plans to changing needs (Baxter et al., 1983).

Staff

There are a total of twelve professional staff (nurses/social workers) and three support staff. TRIMS directly employs thirteen staff members and has a subcontract for the services of one case manager from a local United Way agency and an agreement with Region II Department of Human Resources for the in-kind services of another case manager. Managerial positions include the director, project coordinator, community outreach and development, and case management supervisor.

Clients

The Texas Project for Elders has attempted to provide community-based long-term care services to people 65 and older who are functionally impaired, unable to manage the essential activities of daily living on their own, and lack adequate informal supports. The Elders project has focused on providing services to high-risk elderly in order to prevent their being institutionalized. Client caseload has averaged 320 clients with a range of 305-335 clients in a service area covering more than 710 square miles in Houston and Harris County. The largest referral sources for channeling clients have been family/friends/self (28%), hospitals (21%), and home health agencies (15.2%). (Wilson, 1983.) Criteria for participation have been based on four factors (in addition to client interest):

(1) Impairment. Client must be functionally impaired and assessed to have a minimum of 2 moderate Activities of Daily Living (ADL) impairments, or 3 severe Instrumental Activities of Daily Living (IADL) impairments, or 2 severe IADL impairments and 1 severe ADL impairment.

(2) Need for Service and/or Support. Client must have an unmet need for 2 major personal-care or in-home services that is expected to last 6 months or more; or a fragile informal support system.

(3) Age. Client must be at least 65 years old.

(4) Residence. Client must reside in the service area, or, if institutionalized, must be certified as likely to be discharged to a noninstitutional setting within 3 months.

Organizational Relations

A variety of strategies for interagency collaboration have been essential to the Texas Project for Elders. The project proposal and all service delivery procedures have been developed in collaboration with a working 22-member advisory council of public and private agencies responsible for planning, funding, and delivering long-term care services. The advisory council assisted staff in the planning and development phase and continued to advise staff once the project was operational.

Outreach activities have been used to inform key individuals in the community and to establish linkages with hospitals, home health agencies, public agencies, and other community social service agencies. Strategies and activities have included negotiation of written agreements, inservice presentations, distribution of brochures, use of media, mass mailings of publicity materials, and presentations to community groups and professional associations. Special agreements and contracts have been established with key agencies to streamline referral procedures, eligibility determination, follow-up, and monitoring of service delivery (Wilson, 1984).

Finances

As part of the national channeling demonstration, Texas Project for Elders received a total of four years of funding. Funding was provided in three major categories, with some latitude for shifting funds with appropriate justification. Estimated expenditures were as follows: Site operations: $1,452,821. Funds covered 100% personnel, travel, and all routine operating expenses such as lease and supplies.

Service expansion/gap-filling needs: $116,215. These funds were given to sites solely for the purpose of filling "service gaps" through the purchase of goods and services otherwise unavailable in the community or through a client's benefits (Medicaid/Medicare). Funds were utilized to purchase in-home services, medical equipment, and transportation for project clients.

Automated management information system: $31,250. These funds were awarded for the purpose of developing an automated management information system for client tracking, project management, and fiscal record keeping for service expansion funds. The actual costs included purchase of computer hardware, programming costs, and salary/associated costs of a data clerk.

Contact Information

Contact Nancy Wilson, M.A., Project Director, Texas Project for Elders, 2210 Maroneal, Suite 442, Houston, Texas 77030.

BEST PRACTICE MODEL 4:
WALLINGFORD WELLNESS PROJECT

Background

The Wallingford Wellness Project (WWP) was established in 1979 by the University of Washington School of Social Work with funds provided by the Administration on Aging, United States Department of Health and Human Services. It began as a demonstration and evaluation of a community-based model for improving the health of older people through education and training. The development of WWP was affected by three significant outside influences. WWP was a response to the Surgeon General's 1979 report, *Healthy People,* which emphasized social and economic imperatives for health promotion with older persons. WWP incorporated important features of the 1930s experiment in Peckham, England, which had focused on health promotion and daily health behavior within an intergenerational family and community context. WWP was also influenced by social work practice and the value placed upon empowering participants to acquire the information and skills needed to exercise self-determination.

Objectives

The project has been guided by a strong prevention/health promotion philosophy. A WWP report states,

> The older among us certainly have a right to enjoy the best possible health and hence the highest quality of life for all the years that they live. Further, older people in optimum health, living and working, participating in all aspects of community life constitute a national resource that we can ill afford to waste. Programs and policies which operate to enhance the health and well-being of older persons enhance the health of the nation. (FallCreek & Stam, 1982, p. 4).

The overall goal of WWP has been to improve the health and well-being of project participants through education and training. The four basic objectives have been to (1) design an educational and training program that is appropriate for potential project participants; (2) implement the program; (3) evaluate the impact of the program on participants' lives; and (4) ensure dissemination and perpetuation of the program.

Program

The four core content areas of the WWP educational and behavioral change training programs have included environmental assertiveness, exercise/physical fitness, nutrition, and stress management. The selection of these program components was based primarily on several key studies: McCamy and Presley (1975), Farquhar (1978), *Healthy People* (USDHEW, 1979), and Belloc and Breslow (1972). Classes comprised 10-20 persons and were cofacilitated by two of the five WWP professional staff. After initial trials, three of the classes (physical fitness, stress management, nutrition) were each taught for 7 consecutive weeks, three hours per week, along with environmental assertiveness, which ran for the entire 21 weeks. The contribution of these program components to the prevention/promotion goals is as follows:

Environmental assertiveness included assertiveness training, advocating for a safe and healthy environment, skill development in making and maintaining chosen behavior changes, and promoting self-responsibility for health behaviors.

Exercise emphasized three aspects of physical fitness: increasing individual flexibility and strength; increasing cardiopulmonary fitness by engaging in aerobic activities; and achieving a basic understanding of the physiological effects of exercise.

Nutrition sought to enable participants to make educated choices about diet, and to encourage changes in unhealthy eating habits.

Stress management helped participants learn healthy ways to manage stress in daily life by identifying stress patterns and stressors in their lives and by the use of relaxation techniques (FallCreek & Stam, 1982).

Staff

After six months of staff recruitment and program planning, project personnel consisted of two principal investigators, a project director, project coordinator, project secretary, physician's assistant/health educator, social worker/health educator, research assistant, and two second-year M.S.W. field practicum students. Complementing the staff were 100 persons who contributed more than 1,500 volunteer hours to help create the WWP over a 2.5-year period.

Clients

Classes were age integrated; ages ranged from 13 to 87 years. Data collected for the project's research indicated that the average age of the 90 participants studied was 70 years. The majority (79%) were female. Over half (58%) were married; 42% were widowed, divorced, or single.

Organizational Relations

Relationships with community members and organizations were important to WWP as a key part of its effort to prepare for the day when funding would cease. Two concerns were the focus of relationships: (1) the transfer of program leadership and management from the academic community and program staff to participants and the broader community; and (2) the establishment of an ongoing health promotion program in the Wallingford Senior Center and Senior Services and Centers, Inc., as a foundation for future programs.

Finances

Support was provided by a three-year grant from the Administration on Aging. Approximately $137,000 was awarded each year. Approximately $50,000 of the grant was used for direct services with the remainder allocated to research activities and indirect costs. Clients were not charged to participate in activities although fees were collected to cover cost of materials.

Contact Information

Contact Stephanie FallCreek, D.S.W., Director, The Institute for Gerontological Research and Education (TIGRE), New Mexico State University, Las Cruces, New Mexico 88003. (505) 646-3426.

CONCLUSION

The four best practice models examined in this chapter suggest that planning prevention programs for older persons is a challenging, yet attainable goal. Disease prevention and health promotion programs can be utilized as important strategies for meeting the expanding health and mental health needs of the growing elderly population. Viable and effective prevention-related programs have been developed and implemented by the American Association of Retired Persons and its Widowed Persons Service, Spokane Community Mental Health Center Elderly Services, Texas Research Institute of Mental Sciences and its Texas Project for Elders, and Wallingford Wellness Project. The information and experiences presented about these four programs provide a reference for those involved in creating similar prevention programs. In this concluding section, representatives of these programs suggest a set of ten key action steps necessary in the planning process.

Action 1: Examine Myths on Aging

"Effective program design for health promotion with older people demands that staff and participants alike examine critically the prevalent negative stereotypes of aging which suggest a limited capacity for personal change and community contribution" (FallCreek & Stam, 1982).

Action 2: Define Service Area

"More successful programs seem to be ones which effectively limit their area of involvement. By concentrating on smaller population areas, this gives a group with limited resources the opportunity to be more involved with a particular community" (Prisuta, 1984).

Action 3: Design Effective Recruitment Tools

"The most essential recruitment tools are 'Five Ps': planning, personal contact, phone calls, publicity (media), and presentations. Each of these is important in building credibility, relationships, interest, and finally, personal investment on the part of new participants." These are supplemented by a sixth "P," personal commitment (FallCreek & Stam, 1982).

Action 4: Develop Outreach Strategies

Identify key individuals in the community such as social service agencies, hospitals and other health organizations, churches, social groups, civic associations, and other groups in which older persons participate.

Inform key individuals through distribution of brochures and project posters, use of media (public service announcements, local newspaper ads, and articles), mass mailings of project publicity materials, and presentations to community groups and professional associations (Baldwin, 1983; Morrison, 1983).

Action 5: Employ Experienced and Knowledgeable Staff

"Employ staff with knowledge and skills related to the elderly and the the community and its services. This is important for efficiency and credibility. The educational background of workers can vary, but previous experience working in the community is crucial" (Wilson, 1983).

Skills needed by staff are (1) commitment; (2) tolerance for complex organizational interfacing; (3) communication skills; (4) flexibility, patience, and perseverance; (5) organizational assessment skills; (6) familiarity with service delivery and research perspectives; (7) experience with management, budget, and evaluation; and (8) experience in a liaison-boundary role between hierarchical and nontraditional organizational structures (FallCreek & Stam, 1982).

Action 6: Utilize Program Facilitators

The facilitator's understanding and application of health promotion philosophy, knowledge, and group leadership skills enable prevention programs to work.

The facilitator mediates between each participant and the group by helping the group hear the individual and the individual hear the group. . . . The facilitator must be able to assess each person's capacity to assume leadership within the group in order to continually provide appropriate leadership opportunities for each participant.

Facilitators need to be committed to promoting health in their own lives if they are to effectively share successes, setbacks, and struggles with the participants, and thus provide a model with whom the participants can identify.

Facilitators can also motivate participants to develop. They must also support networks to enhance and maintain behavior change. (FallCreek & Stam, 1982)

Action 7: Build Organizational and Community Relationships

Make initial contacts with other agencies and organizations at the highest level possible. Aim for mutual understanding and the agreement to work together.

Develop linkages with appropriate organizations such as hospitals, home health agencies, community social service agencies, information and referral agencies, and meals on wheels programs.

Negotiate memoranda of understanding or written agreements to facilitate implementation of the relationship.

Continue ongoing contact to maintain successful networking within the informal system (Baldwin, 1983; Morrison, 1983).

Action 8: Foster Volunteer Participation

"Working directly with volunteers is rewarding in that it is often the best way to meet unique client or project needs; however, it is time-consuming. Administration must take this into account when planning staff work loads. Volunteer agencies are valuable and efficient sources of help if their services meet a client's needs. However, this requires establishing and maintaining a working relationship with these agencies. Again, significant staff time must be allotted if mutually supportive relationships are to be created. Working with both volunteer agencies and direct volunteers is recommended" (Corrine, 1983; Texas Department of Human Resources, 1983).

Action 9: Establish Broad Financial Support

It is important that the group face its financial responsibilities from the outset. Although there may be opportunities for a program to be underwritten by one source, such as a foundation or governmental funding agency, this generally is not best for the organization. It tends to eliminate the broad educational and public accounting responsibilities incumbent upon multiple support efforts. Having to attract resources from large numbers of people justifies the organization's efforts to be in the public eye. . . .

Foundations, organizational treasuries, and individuals with substantial resources can be approached by the funding committee to become sponsors and/or provide funds.

Another potential funding resource is a modest direct mail request. Each request should substantiate the need for and anticipate use of funds, the innovative nature of the service, the contributions being made by others (including the volunteers) and the history or interests of the donor that make this a legitimate consideration. (Baldwin & Loewinsohn, 1982)

Action 10: Formulate an Explicit Policy Regarding Client Confidentiality

Guidelines for the types of content and format in a policy regarding confidentiality are as follows:

(1) Keep the names of all persons who contact the program for assistance strictly confidential.

(2) The problems of a client should be discussed between staff and volunteers only when conferring on how to handle a situation or when trying to gain insight into possible future situations.

(3) Never discuss a client in a public setting.

(4) Under no circumstances should the name of the client be given to an agency or other resource without the client's expressed consent.

(5) All agency forms should be turned into the office as soon as the relationship is completed and should not be viewed by anyone other than persons involved in the program.

(6) The major concern should always be in the best interest of the people served. This consideration should guide thinking and action regarding the matter of confidentiality (Baldwin & Loewinsohn, 1982).

References

American Association of Retired Persons. *Introduction to Widowed persons service.* Washington, DC: Widowed Persons Service Program Department, AARP. PF1473 (980).

American Association of Retired Persons. *Widowed persons service fact sheet.* Washington, DC: Widowed Persons Service Program Department, AARP. PF2136 (1082).

Baldwin, E. F. (1983, November). *Interagency cooperation in service delivery.* Paper presented at the 111th Annual Scientific Meeting of the American Public Health Association, Dallas.

Baldwin, L., & Loewinsohn, R. (1982). *Widowed persons service manual.* Washington, DC: Widowed Persons Service Program Department, AARP.

Baxter, R. J., et al. (1983, April). *The planning and implementation of channeling: Early experiences of the national long-term care demonstration.* Princeton, NJ: Mathematica Policy Research. (Research monograph, chapter 2).

Belloc, N., & Breslow, L. (1972). Relationships of physical health status and health practices. *Preventive Medicine, 1,* 409-421.

Binstock, R. H., & Shanas, E. (1976). *Handbook of aging and the social sciences.* New York: Van Nostrand Reinhold.

Busse, E. W., & Blazer, D. G. (1980). *Handbook of geriatric psychiatry.* New York: Van Nostrand Reinhold.

Butler, R., & Lewis M. (1982). *Aging and mental health* (3rd ed.). St. Louis: C. V. Mosby.

Committee on Aging, Group for the Advancement of Psychiatry. (1983, April). *Mental health and aging: Approaches to curriculum development* (Vol. XI, Pub. No. 114). New York: Mental Health Materials Center.

Corrine, J. (1983, November). *Working with informal supports.* Paper presented at the 111th Annual Scientific Meeting of the American Public Health Association, Dallas.

Davis, J. (1983, Spring). Mental well being of elders. Seeking positive solutions. *Generations, 7.*

Dychtwald, K. (Ed.). (1983, Spring). Wellness and health promotion for elders. *Generations, 7*(3).

FallCreek, S., & Mettler M. (1982). *A healthy old age: A sourcebook for health promotion with older adults.* Seattle: Center for Social Welfare Research, School of Social Work, University of Washington.

FallCreek, S., & Stam. S. B. (Eds.). (1982). *The Wallingford wellness project: An innovative health promotion program with older adults.* Seattle: University of Washington.

Farquhar, J. W. (1978). *The American way of life need not be hazardous to your health*. New York: W. W. Norton.

Filner, B., & Williams T. (1981). Health promotion for the elderly. In A. Somers & D. Fabian (Eds.), *The geriatric imperative* (pp. 187-204). New York: Appleton-Century-Crofts.

Gaitz, C., & Varner, R. (1980). Preventive aspects of mental illness in late life. In J. Birren & R. B. Sloane (Eds.), *Handbook of mental health and aging*. Englewood Cliffs, NJ: Prentice-Hall.

Gottesman, L. E. (1981, April). *Client level functions of the long term care demonstration: The basic intervention*. Philadelphia, PA: Temple University Institute on Aging. (paper)

Holstein, M. (1983, Spring). Funding health promotion for elders. *Generations, 7*.

Kessler, M., & Albee, G. W. (1975). Primary prevention. *Annual Review of Psychology, 26*.

Levinson, H. (1972). *Organizational diagnosis*. Cambridge, MA: Harvard University Press.

McCamy, J. C., & Presley, J. (1975). *Human lifestyling: Keeping whole in the 20th century*. New York: Harper & Row.

Morrison, A. (1983, November). *Reaching the "at risk" elder*. Paper presented at the 111th Annual Scientific Meeting of the American Public Health Association, Dallas.

National Research on Aging Planning Panel. (1982). *A national plan for research on aging*. Washington, DC: National Institute on Aging.

Prisuta, R. H. (1984). *Evaluation of the AARP Widowed Persons Service*. Washington, DC: American Association of Retired Persons.

Raschko, R. (1981). *Elderly services – Spokane community mental health center*. Spokane, WA: Spokane Community Mental Health Center Elderly Services.

Raschko, R. (1984). *Spokane case management program*. Spokane, WA: Spokane Community Mental Health Center Elderly Services.

Selby, P., & Schechter, M. (1982). *Aging 2000*. Boston: MTP Press.

Texas Department of Human Resources. (1983). *Program review, Volume 2: Case load buildup, Texas project for elders*. Austin: Author.

U. S. Department of Health and Human Services. (1980). *Promoting health/preventing disease*. Washington, DC: Government Printing Office.

U. S. Senate, Special Committee on Aging. (1982). *Every ninth American*. Washington, DC: Government Printing Office.

USDHEW. (1979). *Healthy people: Report on health promotion and disease prevention*. Public Health Service. Report by Surgeon General. Office of the Assistant Secretary for Health and Surgeon General, Washington, DC.

Warner-Reitz, A., & Mettler, M. M. (1983, Spring). Designing health promotion programs for elders. *Generations, 7*.

White House Conference on Aging. (1981). *Chart book on aging*. Washington, DC.

Wilson, L., Simson, S., & McCaughey, K. (1983). The status of preventive care for the aged: A meta-analysis. In S. Simson, L. Wilson, J. Hermalin, & R. Hess, (Eds.), *Aging and prevention*. New York: Haworth Press.

Wilson, N. L. (1983, November). *Interagency teamwork in community long-term care: An organizational overview*. Paper presented at the 111th Annual Scientific Meeting of the American Public Health Association, Dallas.

Wilson, N. L. (1984). Coordination as a means to improve the long term care delivery system: The Texas long term care channeling demonstration. *GRECC Seminar Series on Aging*. Minneapolis: Veteran's Administration Medical Center.

Wilson, N., et al. (1983, March). *Background on Texas Project for elders*. Houston TX: TRIMS Gerontology Center.

About the Contributors

Sheila H. Akabas is a Professor and the Director of the Center for Social Policy and Practice in the Workplace at the Columbia University School of Social Work. She is currently Project Director of "A Systems Approach to Workers and Their Mental Health" and principal investigator of a research grant "Promoting Rehabilitation Services: EAP's as Effective Advocates" from the National Institute of Handicapped Research. She has authored and coauthored numerous articles and books and has served as consultant to a variety of trade unions, corporations, social, mental health and rehabilitation facilities, and educational institutions.

Stephen E. Goldston is Consultant in Preventive Psychiatry at the Neuropsychiatric Institute, University of California, Los Angeles. He retired from federal service after a lengthy career at the National Institute of Mental Health. During his tenure at NIMH, he participated in the formulation of the national community mental health centers program as a staff associate to President Kennedy's Interagency Committee on Mental Health, in the development of innovative experimental mental health training programs and public health/mental health training projects, and he served as Special Assistant to the NIMH Director, and Director of the Office of Prevention. He has worked in the field of community mental health for the past 27 years. He has published 10 books and monographs, and approximately 40 articles dealing with community mental health, community psychiatry, primary prevention, and public health/mental health. He is a fellow of the American Psychological Association and the American Public Health Association. He has academic appointments in the Department of Psychiatry, University of Maryland; Department of Psychology, University of Vermont; and the Department of Psychiatry and Biobehavioral Sciences, and the School of Social Welfare, University of California, Los Angeles. He is the recipient of the American Psychological Association's 1984 Award for Distinguished Professional Contributions to Public Service, being cited as "the prime architect of the Federal mental health prevention effort."

Jared Hermalin is currently the Executive Director of the Tri-County Council on Alcoholism of Burlington, Camden, & Gloucester Counties, Inc. He was Founder and Director of the Philadelphia Metropolitan Area Self-Help Clearinghouse and Chief of Evaluation of the Consultation & Education/Prevention Service, JFK Community Mental Health/Mental Retardation Center. He received his doctorate from Brown University and his postdoctoral training at Yale. He holds the position of Adjunct Associate Professor in the Department of Mental Health Sciences at Hahnemann University and is credited with initiating the urban field placement program at Swarthmore. He has served as President-Elect and Council member of the Eastern Evaluation Research Society; Representative-at-Large for the National Committee For Mental Health Education; member of an NIMH self-help planning committee; consultant to the National Council of Community Mental Health Centers, the American Lung Association & the Cystic Fibrosis Foundation; and has worked with the Arthritis Foundation. He is an Associate Editor of the *Prevention in Human Services* journal, coeditor of three journal theme issues, reviewer, and author.

Alfred H. Katz received the M.A. with first Class Honours in Psychology, University of New Zealand; M.S.W., New York School of Social Work; and D.S.W., Columbia University (1957). He spent 17 years as a practitioner, administrator, and researcher in family, child welfare and industrial social work before taking a full-time academic position at UCLA, in 1958. Since 1966, he has been Professor of Public Health and Social

Welfare at UCLA, concentrating his research interests on the social-psychological correlates of chronic illness and disability in children and adults, and on the analysis of self-help phenomena. His 8 books and more than 100 professional articles include "Parents of the Handicapped," "Health and the Community," and "Hemophilia: A Study in Hope and Reality." He has been a Visiting Professor at the London School of Economics, the Hebrew University, universities of Copenhagen and Aberdeen, and has lectured at other universities all over the world. He has been a consultant to the World Health Organization, the Ford Foundation and many U.S. and state government agencies. He has been a member of the editorial boards of *Health & Social Work, Prevention in Human Services,* and the new journal *Health Promotion.* He has been an active member and held positions in the American Public Health Association, the National Association of Social Workers, the Association of Voluntary Action Scholars, and other organizations.

Joel Meyers obtained his Ph.D. in Educational and School Psychology from the University of Texas at Austin in 1971. He is Professor and Director of the Programs in School Psychology at the State University of New York at Albany, and he has taught at Temple University, the University of Puerto Rico, and the University of Minnesota, where he also served as Director of the National School Psychology In Service Training Network during 1979-80. He has published over 40 articles, monographs, and book chapters, as well as 4 books concerning mental health consultation as a preventive approach to the delivery of psychological services. In addition, he has worked in the schools as a psychologist delivering preventive services to children, and he has conducted numerous professional workshops on these topics. He belongs to the American Educational Research Association and the American Psychological Association where he holds office as Past-President in the Division of School Psychology. In addition, he coordinated the Spring Hill Symposium on the Future of Psychology in the Schools, which was the first national conference in the field since the Thayer Conference in the 1950s.

Jonathan A. Morell is a research staff member in the Technology Transfer Research Group at the Oak Ridge National Laboratory (ORNL). His interests include the impact of office information technologies and the methodology of evaluation research. He has also been deeply involved in the evaluation of a wide variety of social and human service programs. His activities have been recognized by his election to listing in Who's Who in *Frontier Science and Technology*. He has served as a council member of the Evaluation Research Society, and chairperson of their training committee. He is also a past president of the Eastern Evaluation Research Society. Prior to joining ORNL, he spent a decade as Associate Director of Hahnemann University's graduate program in Evaluation and Applied Social Research and as Professor in the Department of Mental Health Sciences. He is Editor-in-Chief of the journal, *Evaluation and Program Planning,* and author of a textbook, *Program Evaluation in Social Research* (Pergamon Press).

Richard D. Parsons is a graduate of Temple University, where he was awarded both a Master of Arts and Doctorate of Philosophy in Psychology. He is a licensed Psychologist and a Certified School Psychologist. He has given over 300 workshops for parents, educators, and human service professionals on a myriad of topics aimed at facilitating the growth and development of children through direct and consultative services. He has authored or coauthored over 40 professional articles and books. His most recent books include: *Passive Aggressiveness, Counseling Strategies, Developing Consultation Skills,* and *Adolescent in Turmoil: Parents under Stress.* He is currently Professor of Psychology in the Graduate Department of Pastoral Counseling at Neumann College. He maintains a private clinical practice in Media, PA, where he does psychotherapy and provides consultation services to schools and professionals in the tristate area. In addition to professional membership in the American Psychological Association, Eastern Psychological Association, and the National Association of School Psychologists, he has also been named a member of American Men and Women of Science and American Catholic Who's Who.

Sharon Simson is Associate Professor of Mental Health Sciences and Associate Chief of the Section of Geriatric Psychiatry at Hahnemann University School of Medicine in Philadelphia. She was awarded her Ph.D. with distinction by the University of Pennsylvania, where she held a National Institute of Mental Health fellowship. She has been a Fellow in Applied Gerontology of the Gerontological Society of America, a reviewer of discretionary grants for the Administration on Developmental Disabilities, DHHS, and is on the editorial board of *Journal of Evaluation and Program Planning*. She is an organizer with the Widowed Persons Service of the American Association of Retired Persons and was elected delegate to the 1986 AARP Biennial Convention. She is coeditor of *Handbook of Geriatric Emergency Care* (with Drs. L. Wilson and C. Baxter) and *Aging and Prevention* (with Drs. L. Wilson, J. Hermalin, and R. Hess). Her research has focused on aging and mental health, organizational relations, education of health professionals, and long-term care.

Carolyn Swift is Director of the Stone Center for Developmental Services and Studies as Wellesley College. The work of the Stone Center is directed to preventing mental illness and promoting healthy psychological development through research and action projects. She holds a B.A. in Philosophy, and an M.A. in Experimental Psychology, and a Ph.D. in Clinical Psychology from the University of Kansas. In 1980 the National Council of Community Mental Health Centers honored her with an Award for Distinguished Contribution to the field of Consultation, Education and Prevention. She was awarded the Distinguished Practice Award for 1984 from the American Psychological Association's Division of Community Psychology. She has served as a consultant to the National Institute of Mental Health and to mental health centers across the country on issues of prevention. Her publications are in the area of policies and practices related to preventive services in community mental health. A major research focus has been directed to the prevention of sexual child abuse and the prevention of violence against women.

Marshall Swift, a psychologist, is Professor and Director of Prevention Training at Hahnemann Medical University. For 10 years he was the Director of Consultation, Education and Prevention Programs at the John F. Kennedy Community Mental Health/Mental Retardation Center. These organizations collaborated to establish a Preventive Intervention Research Center (PIRC) funded by NIMH of which Dr. Swift is also Associate Director. He received his M.S. and Ph.D. degrees at Syracuse University, B.A. at the State University of New York at Oswego, and did his internship in Clinical Psychology at the Devereux Foundation. He holds the Diplomate from the American Board of Professional Psychology in school psychology. He is research and training consultant to numerous organizations in both public and private sectors, has published over 30 articles, 1 book, and 2 monographs, and given numerous workshops on planning and implementing prevention programs at national and local meetings. He has served as Chair of the Prevention Steering Committee of the National Council of Community Mental Health Centers and currently is the Chair of the Task Force on Psychologists in Applied Settings.

Thomas W. Weirich, Ph.D., is now an Investment Broker with Janney Montgomery Scott in Philadelphia. He was Research Director at the John F. Kennedy CMHC and Clinical Associate Professor at Hahnemann University. With Dr. Swift, he consulted on issues of organizational change and performance from the Consultation Center at Hahnemann.

Laura B. Wilson is currently serving as Associate Professor and Director of the Gerontology Services Administration Program and Executive Director of the Southwest Long Term Care Gerontology Center at the University of Texas Health Science Center at Dallas. The Gerontology Center is one of eleven national long-term care centers and serves DHHS Region VI doing research, education, and service related to long-term care and aging. She has trained in the United States and England in aging, health services, and health planning. Publications in numerous health and aging journals focus on emergency services and long-term care, the impact of DRGs on community-based long-term care, prevention and health of the elderly, and mental health and aging.

NOTES